AF875237

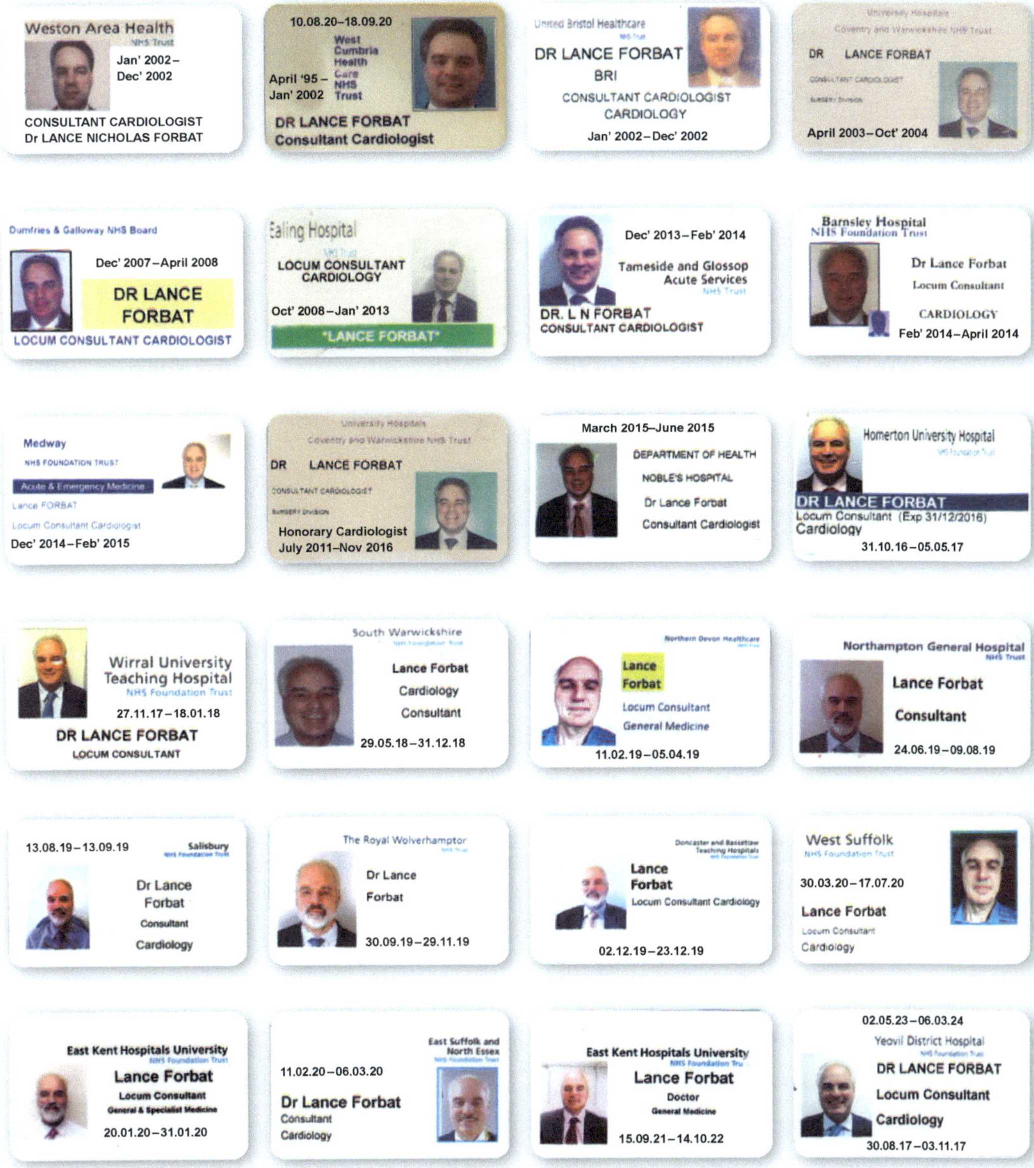
Weston Area Health
NHS Trust
Jan' 2002 – Dec' 2002
CONSULTANT CARDIOLOGIST
Dr LANCE NICHOLAS FORBAT
10.08.20–18.09.20
West Cumbria Health Care NHS Trust
April '95 – Jan' 2002
DR LANCE FORBAT
Consultant Cardiologist
United Bristol Healthcare
DR LANCE FORBAT
BRI
CONSULTANT CARDIOLOGIST
CARDIOLOGY
Jan' 2002 – Dec' 2002
University Hospitals
Coventry and Warwickshire NHS Trust
DR LANCE FORBAT
April 2003 – Oct' 2004
Dumfries & Galloway NHS Board
Dec' 2007 – April 2008
DR LANCE FORBAT
LOCUM CONSULTANT CARDIOLOGIST
Ealing Hospital
LOCUM CONSULTANT CARDIOLOGY
Oct' 2008 – Jan' 2013
"LANCE FORBAT"
Dec' 2013 – Feb' 2014
Tameside and Glossop Acute Services
NHS Trust
DR. L N FORBAT
CONSULTANT CARDIOLOGIST
Barnsley Hospital
NHS Foundation Trust
Dr Lance Forbat
Locum Consultant
CARDIOLOGY
Feb' 2014 – April 2014
Medway
NHS FOUNDATION TRUST
Acute & Emergency Medicine
Lance FORBAT
Locum Consultant Cardiologist
Dec' 2014 – Feb' 2015
University Hospitals
Coventry and Warwickshire NHS Trust
DR LANCE FORBAT
CONSULTANT CARDIOLOGIST
SURGERY DIVISION
Honorary Cardiologist
July 2011–Nov 2016
March 2015–June 2015
DEPARTMENT OF HEALTH
NOBLE'S HOSPITAL
Dr Lance Forbat
Consultant Cardiologist
Homerton University Hospital
DR LANCE FORBAT
Locum Consultant (Exp 31/12/2016)
Cardiology
31.10.16 – 05.05.17
Wirral University Teaching Hospital
NHS Foundation Trust
27.11.17 – 18.01.18
DR LANCE FORBAT
LOCUM CONSULTANT
South Warwickshire
Lance Forbat
Cardiology
Consultant
29.05.18 – 31.12.18
Northern Devon Healthcare
Lance Forbat
Locum Consultant
General Medicine
11.02.19 – 05.04.19
Northampton General Hospital
NHS Trust
Lance Forbat
Consultant
24.06.19 – 09.08.19
13.08.19 – 13.09.19
Salisbury
NHS Foundation Trust
Dr Lance Forbat
Consultant
Cardiology
The Royal Wolverhampton
Dr Lance Forbat
30.09.19 – 29.11.19
Doncaster and Bassetlaw Teaching Hospitals
Lance Forbat
Locum Consultant Cardiology
02.12.19 – 23.12.19
West Suffolk
NHS Foundation Trust
30.03.20 – 17.07.20
Lance Forbat
Locum Consultant
Cardiology
East Kent Hospitals University
NHS Foundation Trust
Lance Forbat
Locum Consultant
General & Specialist Medicine
20.01.20 – 31.01.20
East Suffolk and North Essex
NHS Foundation Trust
11.02.20 – 06.03.20
Dr Lance Forbat
Consultant
Cardiology
East Kent Hospitals University
NHS Foundation Tru
Lance Forbat
Doctor
General Medicine
15.09.21 – 14.10.22
02.05.23 – 06.03.24
Yeovil District Hospital
NHS Foundation Trust
DR LANCE FORBAT
Locum Consultant
Cardiology
30.08.17 – 03.11.17

Lance Forbat is an extra-ordinary person who has led an extra-ordinary life. Dr Forbat has now done the nation the honour of documenting his invaluable, lifelong experiences for us to read and digest in a pithy but amusing manner, bringing in entertaining anecdotes backed up with letters and notes from friends and colleagues. He has drawn a clever, and somewhat sinister, comparison between NHS staff and members of the motorcycle gang, the *Sons of Anarchy*. As someone who has experienced the dark underbelly of the NHS, I find these comparisons highly relatable. Dr Forbat's depth of experience within the NHS is unsurpassed, there is no one else who has worked in as many hospitals all over the UK as a consultant, 31 trusts over 33 years. Dr Forbat is equipped with a razor sharp mind and the bravery required to identify and point out where improvements to services could be made which is clearly in the public interest. He, and his family, paid dearly for his efforts. A robust health service needs staff who can identify issues and bring them to the fore without risk of reprisal. The regulator of NHS trusts, NHS England, needs to encourage trusts to embrace those that raise patient safety concerns. The rest will follow.

Miss Sasha C Burn FRCS(SN)

A unique personal perspective adding to the conversation surrounding NHS whistleblowing, highlighting the immense strain that coming up against a system can place on individuals operating within it. Part memoir, part manifesto *Ungagged – The Sons Of Bevan* will get you thinking about this important issue.

Oenone Forbat

This is a deeply personal account of Dr Forbat's experience raising concerns about patient care within the NHS.

While every case turns on its own facts, the themes explored in this book, including the challenges faced by clinicians who speak up, will resonate with many across healthcare. These experiences must be heard and reflected upon if we are to improve patient safety and organisational culture.

Dr Chris Day

Dr Forbat's experience mirrors that of many others (professionals, managers, leaders, patients, and relatives) who have exposed the 'club culture', poor leadership behaviours, and failure of policy makers to act ethically, which push healthcare organisations into being defensive and avoidant at the expense of patient care. My hope is that this memoir serves as a call to action, and others who are now ungagged speak out. In the words of the late Professor Aidan Halligan, we need to 'run toward problems, especially on a bad day'.

Steve Turner RGN, RMN, Ba(Hons), PGDip ED

I really enjoyed the stories of how training was 'back in the day' and I remember being terrified of the paternoster at St Thomas's. It really made me laugh thinking of you riding it over the top I would never have dared! The trouble that you have taken to ensure that the stories you are telling are factually accurate is a credit to you. What has deeply saddened me is reading how you have moved from place to place, identifying areas that could be improved, but with little support to get the job done. Your resilience and that of your family in all of this is incredible. I hope this tale will encourage others to effect changes within the system and overall be kinder to one another.

Ms Lesley Roberts BSc MBBS MRCOG

Memoir of a Whistleblower in the National Health Service

UNGAGGED

THE SONS OF BEVAN

DR LANCE N FORBAT

First published 2026

Published under licence by Brown Dog Books and
The Self-Publishing Partnership Ltd, 10b Greenway Farm,
Bath Rd, Wick, nr. Bath BS30 5RL, UK

www.selfpublishingpartnership.co.uk

ISBN printed book: 978-1-918428-48-3
ISBN e-book: 978-1-918428-49-0

Cover design by Andrew Prescott
Internal design by Mac Style

Printed and bound in the UK

This book is printed on FSC® certified paper

MIX
Paper | Supporting responsible forestry
FSC® C013604

Memoir of a Whistleblower in the National Health Service

UNGAGGED

THE SONS OF BEVAN

DR LANCE N FORBAT

BROWN DOG BOOKS

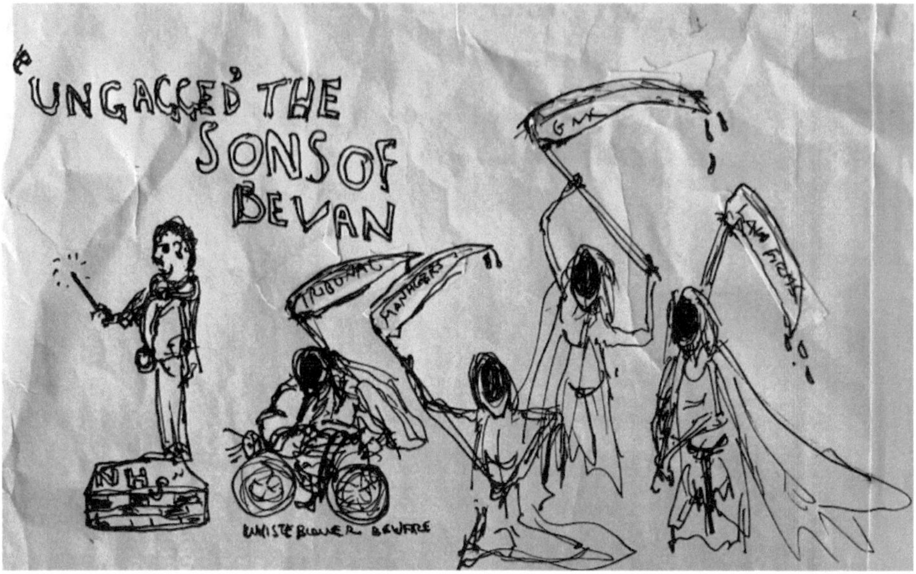

Original sketch in Mont Blanc brown ink

The author drew this in a few minutes with his Mont Blanc pen, with toffee brown ink, whilst watching the NetFlix series, Sons of Anarchy. He saw a parallel between the Charters of the gangs and NHS Trusts, in Aneurin Bevan's NHS. The title comes from the merging of the two in a parallel universe, as depicted here.

When finalising the design of the cover, the author sought permission from the NHS Identity team, as copyright on the NHS logo is all-encompassing. He was told he was not able to use the letters 'NHS' together in any form, so adapted the details taken from the original design above, to avoid infringing copyright.

Dr Lance N. Forbat
BSc(Hons).MD.FRCP.FRCP(Glag)

Foreword for *Ungagged the Sons of Bevan*

All of us have been brought up to tell the truth. Sometimes that truth is painful to hear and even more difficult to process.

In his memoir, *Ungagged the Sons of Bevan,* Dr Lance Forbat has recorded the truth of the events in his medical career that need to be truthfully reported. As the saying goes 'The truth will out', and Lance has made sure that it will out.

Through a series of touching and tragic events experienced through his medical career, Lance describes key moments of his career and includes some of the medical professional hostility that he encountered when he was trying to do the best for his patients. Many doctors still experience the same hostility. This should be unacceptable decades after the NHS and the medical profession should have learnt to do better. If the Bristol Heart Babies Scandal had not taught us all that important lesson, then the Dr Shipman affair and the Mid Staffs debacle with the subsequent Public Inquiry should have guaranteed that we learnt about clinical governance. Sadly, this has not been the case and Dr Forbat's account provides details of episodes where managers, medical professionals and medical managers could all have done better.

It was a senior civil servant who popularised the phrase 'economical with the truth' when explaining the approach of his department in trying to discredit the MI5 Whistleblower Peter Wright. The phrase has since been shamed in popular use but can be used to characterise the approach of medical regulators and some NHS managers in their approach to honest professionals, like Dr Forbat, when they report poor conduct and practice by their colleagues. Dr Forbat is standing up for excellence in patient management and trying to optimise patient outcomes. Failing to respond effectively to Lance's reported examples of poor patient care merely serves to risk the safety of future patients treated by his colleagues. This can cost lives, will cost optimal health and will certainly cost money as the value of care is compromised.

As a Whistleblower myself I understand the turmoil and torment that Lance and his family have endured. Hearing once more that upright professionals bringing examples of poor care to the attention of those who should be dealing with it effectively, but fail dismally, is very saddening. We know that we should do better, and we know that we can do better. To fail to improve is heartbreaking and a betrayal of all those professionals in many specialties and professions who are trying so hard to provide excellent care for their patients.

I hope that this memoir may help the NHS improve.

The sadness is that these stories still need to be told, when we should have learned sooner.

Perhaps the question to be asked is – Why is the NHS such a slow learner?

Stephen Bolsin

Introduction to Sons of Bevan

This book is about the experiences of a doctor whose career crossed paths with bad or misguided individuals who continue to have a disruptive influence on the safe functioning of our NHS.

This narrative is not aimed at the majority of good honest people who comprise this enormous workforce. It however will not exonerate all those good people who turn a blind eye and look the other way when things around them are wrong and where it is in their power to intervene. It is the exposure of the harm done to the service by relatively few who have such an influence in the system. As in all large institutions its survival inevitability trumps the original mission, in the case of our NHS to provide patients safe and free healthcare from cradle to grave.

I identified human characteristics of love, loyalty and people trying (and failing) to find the right way to do the wrong things. The idea crystallised whilst on 'garden leave' watching the series about a turf war between motorbike gangs, presented in the form of a Shakespearean drama about reconciling who you are and learning to live with it.

It centres on the life of a doctor labelled a 'whistleblower' and his recollections from childhood in forming his character to becoming a doctor and how he survived the traumatic onslaught on his life and family, his coping mechanisms that kept him going, maintaining the family unit and his sanity following the rollercoaster of his career for over four and a half decades. I offer some stark solutions.

I dedicate this book to my father and mentor John Egon Forbat (Hungarian immigrant, boyhood evacuee, entrepreneur, author born 26.11.27, died 28.03.18), mother Mary opera singer and mother of five, (born 06.02.29 died 11.12.24 with dementia), my wife, nurse and mother and three daughters who have been passengers on this journey. Thank you for staying the course.

Contents

Prologue

I have 46 years of experience as a doctor that began with the ambition of an 11-year-old boy from Surrey, the son of a Hungarian immigrant family and entrepreneurial spirit, believing in upholding the truth and serving society not the system.

In 2002, soon after publication of the Bristol Royal Infirmary Inquiry report[1] into baby deaths by Professor Ian Kennedy QC, I raised concerns about substandard care in the hospital I recently moved to in the South-West of England, Weston General Hospital, now a merged Trust with the Bristol Royal Infirmary (BRI). The cardiology service had been without a local cardiologist for over six months and was overseen by general physicians with advice from the BRI. Outpatient clinics were run in the interim by an unsupervised staff grade. I was part of the medical on call team and on my ward rounds I observed harm to patients and when no notice or action was taken when raising concerns informally, I submitted online 'Datix' forms which are the accepted way to raise issues. These concerns are reviewed and normally assessed by the relevant clinical lead promptly and shared with those involved for an opportunity to comment and then appropriate learning and any necessary action can be taken to improve care and prevent recurrence. I had no responses, so I continued to submit these daily in increasing numbers. I also came across many cases of concern reviewing patients in my follow-up clinics and the outcome of previous investigations.

The NHS should have an open culture with clinical governance meetings to discuss issues arising from concerns with patient care, yet despite the recent report by Professor Ian Kennedy QC with recommendations, this did not happen and the response was to be told in no uncertain terms by my medical director Dr Trisha Woodhead, to forget about the past and deal with the waiting list. I also had several filing cabinets in my office full cardiac investigations, some over a year-old requiring review with my opinion and my advice to the GPs. I requested the notes for these, as it was essential so I could understand the clinical context. This was refused, there were no electronic records to access the information and so it was not possible to give an informed opinion and advice based on a technician's report. I needed more administrative time in my job plan to deal with the backlog and requested I come out of the general medical rota to manage the cardiology service that had been without a local cardiologist for over six months.

I was unable to do what I knew was required to develop a service from scratch. I have experience from my seven years in Whitehaven. Indeed, before accepting the post at Weston, I made a detailed assessment of the local situation. I made my plans clear in correspondence and meetings with the Medical Director what I needed and how I intended to improve the service. I explained why I needed a period of protected time out of the medical rota to rebuild a safe service. I needed to recruit an experienced cardiac physiologist (I had already head-hunted one from West Cumberland Hospital) to reorganise the department, which in my assessment, was driven by waiting list pressures to maximise throughput at the expense of a quality service.

From the way I was expected to work on instruction from the Medical Director, I felt I had no realistic support. Similarly, I felt little understanding or support from the actions of many of my physician colleagues. I was invariably assigned the weakest junior staff, and apart from the staff grade who helped in clinics (unfortunately, frequently on sick leave) I had no middle grade (junior SHO) above house physician to cover the wards, and when absent, often without provision of locum cover. It was not until I confided in Dr Colin Dyan that I found a colleague who offered understanding and support. In my opinion, because Colin had commitments at both Weston and the BRI, he could appreciate firsthand how different the cardiology practice and the level of support were in the two Trusts. I explained how my job plan was too onerous to manage medicine and cardiology, with the backlog I inherited, the waiting list pressures and, critically, lack of high-quality technical support. The Trust was, in my opinion, unable to offer a safe cardiology service without a consultant cardiologist on site for half a year. Colin was very supportive and he articulated the situation very well in his letter to the Medical Director reproduced here with his consent:

Weston Area Health NHS Trust

26th July 2002

Department of Medicine
Weston General Hospital
Grange Road, Uphill
Weston-super-Mare
Somerset
BS23 4TQ

Tel: 01934 636363
Direct Line: 01934 647174
Dept Fax: 01934 647209

Private & Confidential
Tricia Woodhead
Medical Director
WGH

Dear Tricia

RE: Lance Forbat

I understand from Lance that following his nomination I was to act as an assessor for him in keeping to his current job plan.

Due to time constraints I have not had chance to do this in detail. However since I myself frequently work late to catch on up on paperwork I can confirm that Lance is present later than anyone else in the department often up to 7.00 or 8.00 p.m. or later. I have not been aware of any concerns regarding his clinical competence in Cardiology or General Medicine.

It is my impression that he is obsessional about checking aspects of his patients and this may lead the junior staff to feel that they are being circumscribed.

I am fully aware of the very great backlog in Cardiology and Lance himself has made me aware of this. Like others I have therefore stopping referring anything but the most urgent problems.

Lance has discussed with me several incidences in which he feels that important valve lesions were mis-diagnosed and that the previous cardiac service, although apparently coping in the gap, was actually unreliable. I have no way of verifying this but clearly this could be objectively confirmed.

Lance's insistence on significant private practice, combined with the large workload in Cardiology and his obsessional approach all appear to have contributed to a situation in which there is misunderstandings and mistrust on all sides. The physicians are frustrated that a service apparently that could be managed by one person is now failing but I am fairly sure this was an under-estimate and indeed a second cardiologist was always planned. The trust, not surprisingly, are increasingly anxious about the cardiology backlog and the clinical risks associated with this.

I remain convinced, as I mentioned in a previous e-mail, that the best way to resolve the situation and achieve some success in the cardiology service would be to relieve Lance of his General Medical duties for a significant period of time (e.g. 3 months). If following this he has not managed to make inroads into the cardiology backlog then it would seem appropriate to be concerned about his management of the service. Until then it will tend to be one opinion against another. I am aware that I am in a minority of the physicians in this view and can only speak personally.

I should add that Lance has had some allocations of weaker junior staff (as we all have had at times) which has not helped in his General Medicine and, possibly partly due to his approach, has lost staff in the Cardiac Department who could have been of help. However I believe that he will gradually rebuild these giving him a reasonable opportunity to deliver cardiac goals if he is capable of doing so.

I am writing this letter in an attempt to defuse a situation which I think will otherwise be extremely hurtful on all sides (trust, Dr Forbat, patients) and which may otherwise become a protracted dispute that will go from bad to worse.

Over the last 18 months there has been a lot of additional pressure on the physicians due to unfilled posts, expanding wards and lack of management structure and I am sure this has contributed to a lack of sympathy for this difficult situation. As always I am sure there is failings on all sides here but I am strongly in favour of any route which will be best for patients.

Yours sincerely

Colin M Dayan MA FRCP PhD
Consultant Senior Lecturer

cc

Roger Moyse, Chief Executive
Dr D Wright, Consultant Physician Dr G A
Gould, Consultant Physician
Dr D R Parker, Consultant Gastroenterologist
Dr P Singha!, Consultant Physician
Dr H L Bhakri, Consultant Physician CMD

Sadly, his letter did not change the situation for the better. I only found out why when researching Court hearings related to Weston General in my writing of *Sons of Bevan*. I refer to this in detail in a later chapter.

I was pleasantly surprised, when asking for feedback from my colleagues in Bristol, to learn that Franco Ciulli, a visiting senior lecturer in cardiothoracic surgery at Groby Road Hospital, recalled his time with me when I was cardiology registrar. I met him again on my appointment at Weston General Hospital, when he became a colleague in the cardiothoracic unit in the BRI. He kindly sent me this for my memoir.

> *"Lance Forbat:*
> *Is one of those doctors that come around once in a lifetime. He trained at the court of Prof De Bono in Leicester where I first met him as a registrar and lecturer. Our paths crossed again in Bristol where he was innovating patient care with telemedicine. He was poorly understood by the NHS establishment and eventually was forced to go his own way while attempting to right a system which was archaic and no longer suited modern medicine. His eccentricity masked his knowledge of cardiology and I always found he had the patient's best interest as his paramount concern. He has contributed to helping many cardiology patients nationwide from Cornwall to Glasgow contributing more than most in several lifetimes.*
> *Franco Ciulli"*

I was three months into my new appointment and as the only consultant Cardiologist in the Trust and was taken totally by surprise when the Medical Director informed me there were complaints about my clinical performance. No detailed information was provided and under pressure and with advice from the BMA I agreed to a voluntary review by the NCAA (NCAA, latterly NCS, now Practitioner Performance Advice) prior to my holiday. On my return, I was 'locked out' and I was suspended (put on 'garden leave'). The National Clinical Assessment Association was designed to assess and support 'underperforming' doctors, not lead to their suspension (See NCAA articles on whistleblowers in *Hospital Doctor Magazine*: 'there should be "an open, supportive and learning culture"'). I was not told the reasons for my dismissal at this time, and it was only later in April 2004 the agreed statement was published following the NCAA report and legal arguments (See Statement) giving a completely different view. In my view, my actions qualified as 'protected disclosures', I was a "whistleblower". The Trust, however, following the NCAA report, gave the reason for my dismissal as the 'irretrievable breakdown of trust and confidence'.

The agreed statement in April 2004 (page 200) came after the NCAA report; however, months well before the outcome, the Trust released a statement to the press, published in the local papers. The statements are reproduced below. There is no doubt to me, that this press release, appearing before the NCAA report, damaged my reputation, possibly forever, as they say, 'mud sticks'. I have no doubt the reader, seeing the two statements, will draw their own conclusions and my hope after reading my memoir, my reputation will be restored in the public eye.

The agreed statement in April 2004 (news cutting page 209):

"*The trust and doctor Forbat are pleased to announce that they have settled their differences.*

The trust was pleased to be advised by the NCAA in March 2003 that doctor Forbat is the competent clinician and noted that the workload in the department was too much for a single handed consult furthermore the General Medical Council to whom the trust referred matters decided in summer 2003 that it did not need to take any action.

The trust has appointed 2 consultants to replace Dr Forbat and has apologised for treatment of him and agreed to pay him damages.

Both doctor Forbat and the trust hope that now they have resolved their differences that will be possible for all concerned to put these matters behind them"

Weston & Somerset Mercury 03 January 2003 (news cutting page 204):

> *"A top consultant has been dismissed from Western General Hospital after a catalogue of complaints from colleagues.*
>
> *Doctor Lance Forbat was employed as a consultant physician with the Trust in January 2002 and specialised in cardiology.*
>
> *But after seven months at the hospital doctor Forbat was suspended after a number of concerns about his professional behaviour.*
>
> *The decision was taken after complaints were received from doctors nurses and technicians.*
>
> *A statement from Weston Area Health Trust said staff complained that doctor Forbat failed to prioritise the basic duties on NHS consultant, failed to give clear guidance to junior colleagues and was generally disorganised"*

> *"In view these complaints the Trust has now officially dismissed Dr Forbat*
>
> *Reports on doctor Forbat's dismissal will now be sent to the General Medical Council ensure a proper investigation"*

What is a whistleblower? You are a whistleblower, if as a worker you report certain types of wrongdoing. This will usually be something you've seen at work – though not always. The wrongdoing you disclose must be in the public interest. This means it must affect others, for example, the general public. Another definition of a whistleblower is any individual who provides the right information to the right people. Stated differently, lawful whistleblowing occurs when an individual provides information that they reasonably believe evidences wrongdoing to an authorised recipient. What does whistleblowing mean in health and social care? For example when someone who works for an employer raises a concern about malpractice, risk (for example about patient safety), wrongdoing or possible illegality, which harms, or creates a risk of harm, to people who use the service, colleagues or the wider public? They are acting as a whistleblower. They may not realise this at the time. Emphasis to date has been on creating an environment where staff feel safe to raise concerns but in many healthcare inquiries where there were whistleblowers, the obstacle was not unwillingness of staff to speak out but managerial unwillingness to hear and take action[2].

In the USA they reported a major concern was the fear of reprisals from management by means of 'sham peer review', of which I have been a victim. The American College of Emergency Physicians (ACEP) defines 'sham peer review or malicious peer review…as the abuse of a medical peer review process to attack a doctor for personal or other non-medical reasons'[3]. In those instances, contrived allegations of incompetent or disruptive behaviour and concocted 'sham' peer review are not only retaliatory acts against whistleblowing by hospital administration to elegantly terminate employment, but they are also a career-threatening process for the affected physician. Any adverse privilege action is reported to the National Practitioner Databank (NPDB), which makes it very difficult for the physician to get privileges at any other hospital. Regardless of being adjudicated by a state licensing board, hospitals don't have to remove their adverse action from the NPDB on the practitioner. Kingston et al studied the attitudes of 19 nurses and 14 doctors towards incident reporting. Both professions said simplifying the reporting process would make it easier for them to comply with their professional duty to report. The researchers also suggested that clarification of what constitutes an adverse event or near miss could help improve incident reporting rates.[4]

Healthcare scandals in many countries provide tangible evidence of the significant shortcomings in the protection and support offered to whistleblowers even when they raise legitimate concerns: healthcare organisations frequently disregard such concerns and provide inadequate responses to the issues raised. In some cases, it is clear that senior players seek to ostracise and isolate individuals by undermining their concerns; in extreme cases, healthcare professionals have been disciplined, suspended or reported for misconduct to professional bodies on pretexts derived from a very particular and partisan reading and framing of events. Such experiences are found in the study of 1000 whistleblowers by Public Concern at Work (PCaW)[5]

Dasguota et al[6] reviewed the literature and reported retaliation in seven common types highlighted in studies between 1996 and 2008.

1. Spotlight the whistleblower
2. Manufacture a poor record
3. Threaten them into silence
4. Isolate or humiliate them
6. Prosecute them
7. Eliminate their jobs or paralyse their careers

Debra Jackson et al in their concluding paragraphs state that "*insights into how confidentiality is culturally constructed by nurses and the workplace, and even in the face of poor practice or wrong-doing, whistle blowing can have detrimental consequences for those directly involved. The high personal costs can include individual feelings of distress, marginalization and isolation, and can lead to tarnished reputations and loss of careers. The outcome for the institution, however, may include protection of reputation and risk management of potentially adverse financial outcomes. As revealed by this study, confidentially can be used as a tool to silence individuals and protect the health-care institution, or particular members within the institution, to the detriment of the whistle blower, bystander of a whistle-blowing event or the subject of a whistle blowing complaint.*"[7]

The HCSA definitions on whistleblowing and protected disclosure are from the HCSA's Playbook (see appendix). The term whistleblowing is often used colloquially to describe 'speaking up' and may indicate that there is discomfort being expressed about single or multiple patient safety issues.

A protected disclosure is blowing the whistle in a prescribed fashion, and if done correctly will afford the doctor limited legal protection. A protected disclosure must be shown to have satisfied all the relevant statutory requirements under the Employment Rights Act 1996 (ERA 1996).

This means:

a. there must be a 'qualifying disclosure' under the terms of the ERA 1996
b. it must be in the public interest
c. it must have been made to an appropriate or prescribed person or body.

The terms of ERA 1996 which are relevant to a qualifying disclosure that a doctor might make are that the health and safety of an individual have been, or are likely to be, endangered.

'An appropriate or prescribed person or body' would include your employer, senior management of your organisation, or a prescribed organisation from the official list, which includes the CQC, GMC and NHS England, among others.

A protected disclosure that satisfies ERA 1996 requirements grants some legal protections, including the right not to be dismissed or suffer detriment. These rights are set out in the Public Interest Disclosure Act 1998 (PIDA).

Examples of detriment would be being overlooked for training opportunities or being subjected to spurious disciplinary investigations. However, employers may also claim that the concern you raised was not actually a protected disclosure, and that you are therefore not protected.

Although PIDA grants some legal protections over whistleblowers, it is not always possible to prove that an individual has been dismissed or suffered detriment principally due to a protected disclosure.

Prior to the NCAA report (which dismissed claims of incompetence) being finalised, but not soon enough for the CEO of this Trust, who appeared unable to wait (See article "NCAA stands by decision not to sacrifice care for speed" Talking Points: *Hospital Doctor Magazine* 20 February 2003) I was 'sacked' one week before my first year of employment was up. (See *The Weston & Somerset Mercury* "Top consultant dismissed"). I believe the Trust got rid of me quickly so they could avoid the embarrassment of having to deal with an employee who could be exonerated by the NCAA. To continue practicing as a doctor, I felt I had no option but to settle which included a 'gagging clause', meaning I could not disclose everything. Gagging clauses in respect of protected disclosures are not lawful, but the law around protected disclosures is not fit for purpose in my view. I truly believe I was sacked because of the concerns I raised but I would have had to go to court to prove that and that would have had a detrimental effect on my career, finances and family. I have decided after 24 years and since gagging clauses are no longer allowed, it is time I become 'un-gagged' and the seeds of this book were sown.

My inspiration to finally tell my story and in this form of a narrative, came to me and was prompted while watching *Sons of Anarchy* during a period of unemployment as a result of a GMC investigation with associated restrictions on practice known as conditions. The characters in this account are real. They include those in the roles of the chief executive, medical director, clinical lead, consultant colleagues, medical staffing, finance department, medical indemnity insurer, the GMC, lawyers and my family. Most in the working environment are honest hard-working reliable colleagues I hoped could be trusted. This was to be put to the test. There are however those who behave in a way that mirror personalities and characteristics of villains in *Sons of Anarchy* in which our society is reflected here, as the tapestry of human nature, tribalism, poor relationships, greed, power, compassion, human fallibility and more. The good in individuals is crushed by the system. Accountability is lacking as all efforts of the institution are directed towards maintaining the status quo. I refer to the players here as "*The Sons of Bevan*".

Glossary of Terms

NHS Trust	Legal entity
Trust Chairman	Board of governors overseeing quality
Chief Executive Officer (CEO)	Where the buck stops
Medical Director	Accountable to the CEO
Clinical Lead	Departmental responsibility
Consultant	Specialist 'head of firm'
Trainee	Supervised junior
Medical Student	Medical school deanery responsible
Patient and liaison service (PALS)	Intermediary patient advocate
Freedom to Speak Up Guardian	Advocate for employees
Medical Staffing	Workforce management
Occupational Health	Workforce health
Finance Department	Budgetary responsibility
Health Minister	Supreme authority
Parliament	Holds the health minister to account
Strategic Health Authority (SHA)	Previously Local Health Authority (LHA)

Commissioning Groups	General Practitioner purchasers
Whistleblower	Anyone raising a (qualified) concern
BMA	British Medical Association - Doctors union
HCSA	Hospital Consultants Specialist Association
Nurses	SRN, State Registered. SEN, State Enrolled
HCA	Health care assistant
Patients	Now powerful consumers
GMC	General Medical council, doctors' regulatory body

Cast List: *Sons of Anarchy*

This book is based on actual events but in certain cases I have compared individuals, groups, organisations and incidents with characters from the fictional TV series, *Sons of Anarchy*. This is done for dramatic purposes only and it is not intended that real persons resemble the fictional characters in every way. I observed some of the characteristics embodied by the players in *Sons of Anarchy*, that I was confronted with in the NHS.

Some of these characters were destined to die as a result of war between the Charters, and others at the hands of family members. You may wish to assign different characters from the Sons of Anarchy, to players in my story. If you have experience as a whistleblower, consider casting players in your personal parallel universe.

Chief Executive Officer *Clay Morrow* The President of SAMCRO (Sons of Anarchy Motorcycle Club, Redwood Original - Weston Trust) is a vigilante who does everything in his power to ensure the drug dealers and the rapist stay out of his town.

Medical director *Jax Teller Vice president,* is conflicted between wanting to maintain the longevity of the organisation and his desire to become a law-abiding family man while still living up to his father's legacy and plans, and forms the central conflict of the series.

Consultant A *Tig Trager* the club's most violent member and very loyal to the president. Chibs Telford is nicknamed "Chibs" because of his facial scars ("Chibs" is slang for "street blade" or a stabbing weapon). The scars on his face are real scars Flanagan received in a bar scuffle where his attackers branded him with the "Glasgow smile".

Consultant B *David Hale* is an honest policeman who wants to rid the town of SAMCRO.

Jacob Hale Jr *(Clinical Lead B)* is the older brother of Deputy Chief of Police David Hale and local political bigwig with property interests in the town of Charming.

Chibs Telford, *(Senior manager)* named because of his facial scars (Chibs is Scots slang for 'street blade' or stabbing weapon) has a genuine 'Glasgow Smile', is also very close to Clay.

Medical Secretary A *Tara Knowles* Jax Teller's high-school sweetheart, a paediatric resident at the local hospital, St Thomas's. She marries Jax and has his second son.

Medical Secretary B Wendy Case was a meth addict during her pregnancy, which nearly killed Abel, born premature and first son of Jax.

Consultant C *Kipp Epps* A surprisingly formidable fighter, also a vegetarian. Known also as "Half Sack" having lost a testicle in action in the Iraq war.

Cardiothoracic surgeon *Lee Toric* had a long list of misconduct violations, excessive force, intimidation and racial profiling.

Patient and liaison service (PALS) *Wayne Unser* plans to retire, surrendering his post to Deputy Chief of Police David Hale, but is forced to resume his duties when Hale is killed in a hit and run/drive-by at the beginning of season three. SAMCRO can no longer maintain their deal with the Charming Police Department, where the police would look the other way on SAMCRO's activities in exchange for keeping violence out of Charming.

Freedom to speak up guardian *Piney Winston* Vietnam Vet, felt ostracised by the same society he had just risked his life for. He and Jax's father John Teller, were the founders of SAMCRO.

Medical Staffing *Gemma Teller* She is unapologetic about the lengths she'll go to in order to protect the club and is beloved by all of its members

Finance department *Chuck Marston* Chuck proved to be rather paranoid and also afflicted with compulsive masturbation disorder that reared itself at inopportune times. Chuck led them to the money, but SAMCRO was upset when it was revealed that the money was counterfeit.

Health Minister *Lee Toric* had a long list of misconduct violations, excessive force, intimidation and racial profiling.

Deputy Chief *David Hale Jr.* even-tempered (an uncommon trait among his club-mates), businessman and older brother of the late Deputy Chief David Hale, determined to remove SAMCRO from Charming.

Nurses *Harry (Opie) Winston* best friend of Jax since childhood. Opie's family has difficulty making ends meet, which contributes to Opie's decision to resume illegal activity with SAMCRO.

Whistleblowers *Juice Ortiz* is known for his intelligence and technical skills, often serving as the club's main tech expert. He is proficient at computer hacking and surveillance, which proves valuable in various operations. Despite his capabilities, Juice often struggles with feelings of inadequacy and a desire to belong. He becomes involved in various conflicts, secrets, and dangerous situations. He grapples with personal demons and the consequences of his actions, often finding himself caught between loyalty to his brothers and his own survival. His journey showcases the challenges of loyalty, identity, and the consequences of one's choices in a world as intense and dangerous as that of the motorcycle club.

'Reaper Table' *(Boardroom)* As in this narrative, doctors who are struck off by the GMC and patients who die, are collateral damage due to actions of the Trusts. *(Scene – Clay addressing the members page 178).*

Patients	Residents of Charming
NHS trusts	The Charter SAMCRO and others
GMC	FBI/ATF
Medical Indemnity (MPS/MDU/Euna etc)	Solicitors and barristers

Chapter 1

Treading Water May – July 2021

While writing this I have just spent the last two weeks waiting, watching my first Netflix series, broken when necessary by walking Mary our Cockerpoo, replacing windowsills, painting windows or clearing the garden. I had spent over a year working away from home during the week as a locum consultant cardiologist, which meant jobs just piled up. As I begin writing this story, I have not had income for the last six weeks, surviving on savings deferred for tax and other debts. I feel deflated, unwanted, angry, betrayed and powerless. I have visceral memories of my experience at Weston General.

How did a boy's dream of a successful career as a doctor go 'off-piste' and would I get back on course? I take you back to 1995 when general practices were Fund Holders. This meant money followed patients to where services were best. The entrepreneurial spirit of my father was well absorbed into my psyche and driven by a personality and determination honed by years of climbing the medical career ladder. It made a perfect fit for my skill set and a rewarding seven years, five single-handed, in setting up a highly respected cardiology department in Whitehaven in the deprived North West Cumbria. With my technical team, we set up Ethernet ports for hospital-wide reporting of cardiac ultrasound studies (echocardiograms) and High Tech Link lines across the Pennines to send images to cardiothoracic centres, The Freeman Hospital, Newcastle and South Cleveland , Middlesbrough.

I was empowered and at last could use my knowledge, skills and vision to build a cardiology service in this remote place.

It was far from family roots in the south with children growing up and one boarding in Millfield on a scholarship, and eventually these circumstances precipitated our move to be near to our family ties. This move was the start of where I ended up today and forms the backdrop in which this narrative unfolds.

THE WEST CUMBERLAND

Times & Star

WEST CUMBERLAND JOURNAL Friday, April 21, 1995

Page 2

New heart specialist

WEST Cumbria NHS Health Care Trust has appointed its first consultant cardiologist.

His prime objective is to launch a comprehensive cardiology assessment and treatment service.

Dr Lance Forbat, 39, takes up his appointment at the West Cumberland Hospital, Whitehaven, on Monday and says he welcomes the challenge in an area where the incidence of heart disease is one of the highest in the northern region, and one of the biggest causes of premature death in West Cumbria.

Married with three young daughters, Dr Forbat trained at St Thomas's Hospital, London.

After qualifying he worked in a number of hospitals in and around the capital. He then spent time working on a special medical project in Saudi Arabia, before returning to the UK to specialise in cardiology.

During the last ten years he has worked as a consultant locum in Truro hospital, Cornwall, Musgrave Park hospital in Taunton, and for the past year at Good Hope Hospital NHS Trust in Sutton Coldfield.

Lab helps heart patients

WEST Cumbrian heart patients will benefit from a new laboratory to be installed at the West Cumberland Hospital in Whitehaven.

The purpose-built mobile catheter laboratory will be able to perform angiogram tests - X-rays of the heart - a valuable diagnostic tool in treating heart patients.

Dr Lance Forbat said: "Patients are treated under local anaesthetic and the test allows us to have a moving picture of blood flow through the heart.

"We hope that the health authority will eventually have a catheter laboratory installed on site. It is a very useful tool in helping to establish what type of treatment is appropriate to heart patients."

The laboratory has been funded by the local charity, West Cumbria Heart and Angina Support Group, as a direct result of sponsorship from the radioactive waste disposal company, Nirex.

The West Cumbria Heart and Angina Support Group was set up in 1993 to provide moral and financial help to the Coronary Care Unit of the West Cumberland Hospital.

It is the only heart and angina charity to dedicate all its fundraising for the benefit of West Cumbria and has so far raised around £60,000.

THURSDAY JUNE 1, 1995 ISSUE NO. 792

West Cumbrian

Gazette

News & Star / Thursday, June 1, 1995

Lab on the road to healthier hearts

HEART patients will benefit from a purpose-built mobile laboratory based at West Cumberland Hospital.

The 40ft laboratory is designed to carry out angiogram heart operations — to search for possible artery blockages — without patients travelling to Newcastle.

Financed by West Cumbria Heart and Angina Support Group and Nirex, the lab will make monthly visits to the hospital to help eventually treat more than 300 patients a year.

Dr Lance Forbat, new resident cardiologist, said the laboratory — which will cost £5,000 for each visit — was "a major step forward".

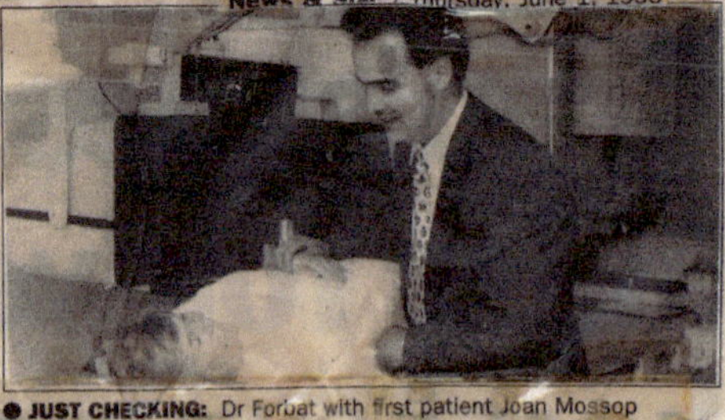

● **JUST CHECKING:** Dr Forbat with first patient Joan Mossop

Prior to the GMC investigation and a further four months out of work, I was a locum cardiologist in a small hospital in West Wales where I found a hospital not too dissimilar to my first appointment. There was difficulty in recruiting consultants, not every major speciality was available onsite

Hi-tech link for heart patients

THE WEST Cumberland Hospital is the first in the UK - and possibly the world - to provide a computer-based remote diagnostic system for people with heart problems.

The £42,000 equipment, allows instant links between Whitehaven and specialist cardiologists elsewhere. It means vital decisions can be made in minutes rather than hours or days.

The equipment, which has been bought with funding from the West Cumbria Heart and Angina Support Group, will start sending images to its main referral hospitals at Newcastle and South Cleveland as well as Glasgow Children's Hospital in the next month.

Sound words

SIR — Re: Cardiothoracic Services in Cumbria "Grasping the Nettle", Ron Copland, referred to his vision of Cardiothoracic services in Cumbria (*The Whitehaven News 25.11.99*).

His sound comments are based on a consultation document from Eugene Milne, Consultant in Public Health Medicine Newcastle and North Tynside Health Authority. Submissions were invited from any individual or agency with an interest.

The imminent publication of the National Service Framework for Coronary Heart Disease emphasised the need for a structured approach to planning services. Options suggested included a). Enlargement of the Freeman, b). Expansion of alternative (out of district and private) providers, c). Use of local hospitals for investigation and basic revascularisations.

The emphasis was on what can be done. A sub-regional cardiothoracic unit is a viable option for the remote 318,000 population of North Cumbria. If the public share this vision then they need the determination to secure the appropriate funding so that "unfilled promises be swept aside".

LANCE FORBAT,
BSC (HONS), MD, FRCP.
Consultant Cardiologist, WCHC NHS Trust.

THE WHITEHAVEN NEW[S]

COMMERCE AGRICULTURE

[THUR]SDAY, OCTOBER 25, 2001

SERVING THE COMMUNITY SINCE 1852

Dismay as heart specialist resigns

by Dave Siddall

THE resignation of the leading heart specialist at Whitehaven's West Cumberland Hospital has dismayed a charity which tirelessly fundraises to help tackle the area's heart disease crisis.

Dr Lance Forbat, who has been at the West Cumberland Hospital for six years, handed in his resignation last week.

His shock move - for personal reasons - means the area has only one cardiologist, Dr Katherine Wilmer.

Ronnie Copeland, founder of the West Cumbria Heart and Angina Support Group which has injected more than £200,000 into boosting cardiology, says the area needs three cardiologists to deal with the case load.

"The amount of work this man [Dr Forbat] has put in has been phenomenal.

"One cardiologist alone would not suffice for an area like West Cumbria which, according to all the statistics, is riddled with heart disease.

"I was shocked to learn of the resignation of Lance Forbat.

"In the first year we helped enable Dr Forbat to advance his work by funding a visiting mobile laboratory to the tune of £82,000.

"The situation with heart disease case loads in West Cumbria is such that we need three cardiologists.

"The situation needs to be seriously addressed both by the hospital trust and by our support group."

Adrian Pattinson, chairman of the West Cumbria Open Heart Surgery Club, said he was devastated by the resignation.

"I am absolutely gutted. We were just getting things together with a second cardiologist, Kate Wilmer, and things were starting to get going.

"It's going to be a blow to West Cumbria. The committee feels knocked sideways."

Nick Wood, chief executive of the North Cumbria Acute Hospitals Trust, said Dr Forbat "would leave behind a fantastic legacy of improved heart services and so it should be easier to recruit a new consultant".

"Dr Forbat, who has accepted a post in Weston-Super-Mare, pioneered a revolutionary mobile angiogram service in West Cumbria which means patients are tested in a matter of hours rather than weeks," he said.

Two years ago, Dr Forbat was the only cardiologist working full-time at the hospital and patients had to wait up to 10 months to see him. Mr Wood is confident that will not happen again.

"There is far more movement of staff than there ever used to be and although we are disappointed Dr Forbat is leaving, it is a natural move for him," he said.

Dr Forbat leaves in January. Advertisements are being prepared to find a replacement.

and it was at the peak of the second wave of COVID-19. I witnessed adequate PPE was fortunately available for medical and nursing staff, however, healthcare assistants were left unprotected despite spending as long or longer than the clinical staff in contact with patients, usually in confined areas with no ventilation, so aerosols of virus particles could gather. When I went in to assess patients in closed patient bays, I was fully protected with a fresh FP3 mask, visor, surgical gown and gloves, however the healthcare assistants wore plastic aprons and standard surgical masks *(which provide no protection from Covid-19).* The hospital management, as is typically the case, was led by a senior nurse, often with no medical equivalent in the hierarchy.

I was able to contribute significantly to the local service as well as maintaining my interventional skills in coronary angiography and pacemaker insertion at other hospitals in the network. Clive Weston is a colleague who I had known over the years from meetings at the British Cardiovascular Society but had never worked with him. He was the Lead for Cardiology in South Wales. I was open and fully transparent with him about my situation leading up to this locum post.

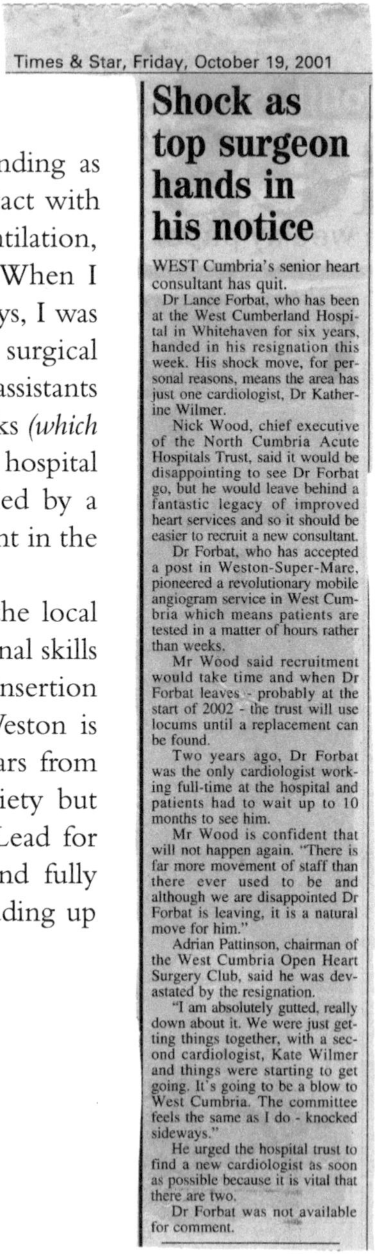

Times & Star, Friday, October 19, 2001

Shock as top surgeon hands in his notice

WEST Cumbria's senior heart consultant has quit.

Dr Lance Forbat, who has been at the West Cumberland Hospital in Whitehaven for six years, handed in his resignation this week. His shock move, for personal reasons, means the area has just one cardiologist, Dr Katherine Wilmer.

Nick Wood, chief executive of the North Cumbria Acute Hospitals Trust, said it would be disappointing to see Dr Forbat go, but he would leave behind a fantastic legacy of improved heart services and so it should be easier to recruit a new consultant.

Dr Forbat, who has accepted a post in Weston-Super-Mare, pioneered a revolutionary mobile angiogram service in West Cumbria which means patients are tested in a matter of hours rather than weeks.

Mr Wood said recruitment would take time and when Dr Forbat leaves - probably at the start of 2002 - the trust will use locums until a replacement can be found.

Two years ago, Dr Forbat was the only cardiologist working full-time at the hospital and patients had to wait up to 10 months to see him.

Mr Wood is confident that will not happen again. "There is far more movement of staff than there ever used to be and although we are disappointed Dr Forbat is leaving, it is a natural move for him."

Adrian Pattinson, chairman of the West Cumbria Open Heart Surgery Club, said he was devastated by the resignation.

"I am absolutely gutted, really down about it. We were just getting things together, with a second cardiologist, Kate Wilmer and things were starting to get going. It's going to be a blow to West Cumbria. The committee feels the same as I do - knocked sideways."

He urged the hospital trust to find a new cardiologist as soon as possible because it is vital that there are two.

Dr Forbat was not available for comment.

08.04.21 Clive Weston - (Hywel Dda UHB - Locum Consultant Acute Physician)

During our last couple of meetings, I have offered to send you a short summary or review of your activity during the months that you have been practicing as a cardiologist (and general physician) within the Health Board. You mentioned that this would prove useful for you at future appraisals. Apologies that I am a little slow in providing you with feedback.

I am doing this in my role as Clinical Lead for Cardiology within Hywel Dda University Health Board. Within the Health Board you have been asked to perform Consultant duties (as a locum) at Withybush General Hospital, Haverfordwest. Additionally, we have been able to arrange some sessions of cardiology procedures at neighbouring hospitals - pacing at Glangwili General Hospital, Carmarthen, and coronary angiography at Prince Philip Hospital, Llanelli.

Obviously, while I have taken opportunities to 'back fill' your clinical duties at Withybush during some of these procedural sessions and so have some indirect insights into your clinical 'modus operandi', these few comments are not based on daily personal or professional interactions. Certainly they are augmented by, or are a summary of, various unsolicited reports from colleagues with whom you have more regular contact.

The first thing to report is that you have made a positive contribution to the cardiology service in Haverfordwest. I know that the senior nursing staff and your substantive consultant colleague are happy with your involvement in the care of patients on the cardiac ward, the latter expressing a wish that you continue to practice in the hospital beyond the planned end date of your locum contract. It is encouraging that the hospital managers have indeed extended that contract. They would not have done so were there any concerns about your fitness to practice or any discontent with your service.

Unlike some clinicians who perform locum duties and so have little interest and involvement in clinical or strategic developments, you have demonstrated a disposition to innovate. You have sought to introduce new systems of documentation in the management of patients, most notably in your introduction of charts for the management of heart failure and problem lists for inpatients. While these have been used with varying degrees of accuracy and completeness by others, and you have to remember that some will take to these more easily and readily than others - what is obvious or 'second nature' to you will not be so to others - when used as they are designed to be used they do appear to be helpful in providing efficient and safe care. I was particularly pleased to see the supportive comments regarding the 'diuretic/ weight' documentation from one of our community heart failure nurses who had taken on the care of one of your patients upon their discharge. [I also note that you were prepared rapidly to respond to her questions about the continuing care of the patient].

I should also point to another disposition - namely a tendency actively to attempt to solve problems. An example of this is your recent dogged 'detective work' in trying to understand the transport/ambulance system whereby patients are prioritised for interhospital transfer. Rather than simply accepting that timely transport could not be provided you set out to find out why, and to educate others as to what might need to be done in future. At this point, and not specific to the issue of ambulance transport, I would issue a word of caution - and that is that some inefficiencies in the NHS reflect inadequate resources, a mismatch of supply to meet demand. When we find a way of prioritising our own patients we often unwittingly disadvantage others. We need to continue to advocate for our own patients and our own service while also reflecting on the needs and feelings of other colleagues and other services - it's difficult.

Lastly, to let you know that I appreciate the difficulty of a 'new boy' coming into established teams in the pacing theatre or the cath lab - every action that differs from their usual practice is a potential source of loss of trust and confidence. One feels 'on display' and vulnerable. The need to begin 'under the supervision' of another consultant, while a necessary requirement for 'patient safety', is potentially demeaning. You have moved beyond this to performing these procedures independently.

So, if this were a school report, I believe that we would underplay things by saying that you can be 'content' with your 'progress'. You have forged good relationships with work colleagues, you have demonstrated an interest in innovation and a commitment to your patients, and a willingness to educate junior doctors. Remember to continue to reflect upon the effects of your innovations and your advocacy on others, who may have differing (rather than opposing) priorities and objectives. Keep at it!

Best wishes,

Clive Weston

Clinical Lead, Cardiology.

The initial three-month contract was extended to over six months, however the unfolding of events of two years passed culminated on the 11th of May in this locum ending abruptly. How this came about will be dealt with in Chapter 7. It took four months and 40 failed applications before I could find any work in the NHS, with no private practice and my modest medicolegal practice, decimated.

Healthcare Inspectorate Wales (HIW). The latest HIW inspection of Withybush General Hospital took place in 2019, and the overall rating given was "Adequate." To improve, such as ensuring that there were enough staff with the right skills to provide safe and effective care, improving the management of patient records, and addressing issues with the cleanliness and maintenance of the hospital.

I wrote chapters 1–6 in this period of four months without work and chapters 7–12 were written in a further six-month break waiting for the GMC to conclude its investigation. I was filling in time doing those things usually left to weekends, now seven days a week. Telling my wife the bad news was hard, telling my daughters, even harder. I put off the day as this bombshell landed on my wife's birthday and shortly after Father's Day celebrations and announcement of a new grandchild on the way. All my financial commitments, including servicing debts dating back over 20 years, had to be managed with no money coming in and no way of predicting when it would restart. Imagine the stress on me and my family and how I was feeling. I am treading on water, looking out to shore to see if there is a safe place to land. There is no lighthouse to guide me, no buoys to hang onto as I build my own raft to safety.

Chapter 2

The Childhood Ambition 1967

As one of five children my primary school years included free school milk, free school dinners and walking to school each day. School was something I looked forward to and I was drawn to subjects that stimulated my imagination. I enjoyed sports and taking part in teams and whilst I was not a gifted sportsman regularly made the team. I took the 11 plus exam the week my grandfather died and failed dismally, at least that's what I thought. My parents believing I deserved better persuaded a local grammar school to take me on.

At 11 years old I knew I wanted to be a doctor. I cannot think of my reason at the time or why it was so clear in my mind to be a doctor, I just knew this is what I wanted to be. I had no immediate family experience of medical careers and only learned later in growing up that my father's brother (our 'Uncle Andrew') was an anaesthetist and their father when in Hungary did start studying medicine, but after they emigrated to the United Kingdom he could not get any place.

In my first year, I wore shorts I had in primary school when other boys had long trousers and my voice broke later than my peers. Despite this, my determination and character shone through. I was the butt of some bullying as a result and on one memorable occasion after being spat on in the ear, I decked the offending bully and was never troubled again. To my surprise and delight I was appointed Villiers Housemaster and in the sixth form became Deputy Head Boy. I took up archery, initially in my back garden with a cheap fibreglass recurve bow, wooden arrows and straw boss. Having decided the garden was too short I found a strip of land beside a road near our house in Surrey and set up my target and began shooting an end of arrows. Not long after this first adventure a car pulled up and a tall, bearded man got out and said, "you shouldn't really be shooting here, but I belong to an archery club" and he invited me to join. Like many boys I had an imagination and Robin Hood featured highly as did my other boyhood hero James Bond and his Aston Martin. I've never lost my desire to own my own Aston Martin.

I joined the Cubs along with my brother and following the example of my father, we progressed to the Sea Scouts and our world opened up with the challenges ahead. We took to the water and became skilled oarsmen and sailors. I took part in the Duke of Edinburgh's award scheme with my brother, attaining bronze, silver and gold and met Prince Philip at the award ceremony and achieved the status of Assistant Scout leader before leaving to study medicine at St Thomas's Hospital Medical School. The story that follows begins with 13 years of training and study, attaining a first-class Physiology degree, an MD, negotiating jobs from preregistration house officer to the first cardiologist and physician in Whitehaven, a remote hospital of West Cumberland.

In 1994, halfway through a Sea Scout camp in the Medway Estuary, I took a day out to visit the local accident and emergency department in Medway Hospital hoping to get a taste of what my medical student career might bring me. I was in my pre-clinical year at St Thomas's and full of excitement about seeing what practical use my anatomy and physiology would bring. I could not resist a closer look. I had in my mind's eye how I would be a great doctor, imagining I might discover some new condition or invent a new treatment. My family was non-medical (apart from an uncle who was an anaesthetist in the USA). I was used to the way my father an engineer, businessman and entrepreneur was always looking to invent or search new markets to meet new targets and support his five children, all born within seven years. My father was one of two brothers whose parents were economic migrants from Budapest, coming to the UK when he was seven years old. He spoke Hungarian and German and no English and wore a velvet suit and shoes with a pageboy haircut. Dad was bullied initially but rapidly integrated and achieved high grades in his matriculation before achieving an engineering degree. He joined Vickers as an aeronautical engineer and later went into business as a salesman, travelling abroad several weeks a year for large companies before taking on the mantle of Managing

Director of his first company. In my long vacations I was a relief milkman for Job's Dairy, my first real taste of dealing with the public in all its variety. I also learned about money and how difficult it can be to balance the kitty to the last penny at the end of the milk round. A forgotten loaf charged or extra pint dropped not on the van on return to the depot came out of my wages. I was getting up at 04.00 and cycling to the depot for my round. I would shadow a milkman for a few days, then be given the books for the round I was taking on. My first duty was loading the electric milk float with crates of 20 pints of milk. Sometimes these were loaded with a forklift truck, more often I would go to the large walk-in fridge and lift two or three crates onto my van. The groceries were loaded in the cupboard at the rear. There was no lock on the doors. I wore a leather money bag or satchel over one shoulder. It had a couple of dividers to which I added a 'float' of change and notes in preparation for giving change to customers. On occasions when taking on a round there were conflicts of conscience, as on some rounds I soon learned that the absent milkman was running a fiddle with the occasional unwary customer by adding a pint or a loaf of bread on the weekly bill. Some would have different orders on different days of the week and not notice as long as the amount charged was consistent. I had to work out a way to not overcharge without shopping the regular milkman. On some rounds the milkman had a boy as a runner and occasionally I inherited them, running the milk and any groceries on the doorstep, as I shouted out the next set of orders (e.g 2 silver, 1 red, eggs, 3 silver, 2 gold, 1 loaf; no milk as on holiday, 3 red 1 brown loaf – not Wednesdays) whilst bringing the van to a stop. My rounds were initially local to me in Surrey but one summer I was needed in Hanwell and provided with a loan car, a navy blue 2.0 litre Ford Cortina, quite a nippy car for the time. On one round I regularly stopped to deliver adjacent to Heathrow airport and had the exciting spectacle of watching Concorde take off and land. Hanwell was a rough neighbourhood, and I now regret that I took on a boy from the locality as my runner. I was towards the last road on one of my rounds but without a runner and my head down in the cab, reading the book for the next few drops. 'Bang' I was hit in the face. Dazed, instinctively I lashed out with both arms just managing to remain upright in the cab. Then it was over, maybe there were two of them, I had the realisation it might be one of the 'runners' I had helping on the van or their acquaintances. I felt blood on my lip and then a sharp edge to one of my top front teeth that I later saw was half gone. I checked my money bag dipping in with my left hand and it was empty bar a few coins at the bottom. All my takings for the day, maybe a couple of hundred pounds, had been stolen. In my right hand I was clutching something soft and when I opened my palm there was a blue and green Pompom hat and a large clump of brown locks fell to the cab floor. Good, I thought, that must have hurt whoever owned it! There were no mobile phones in those days to call the police or contact the depot, so I drove back the last stretch rather sore and relayed the scenario to the office manager. The police were informed but nothing came of it and for the next week I was on desk duties in the Depot, resuming rounds once I felt fully recovered.

It is from this backdrop that I entered the strange new world of medicine. It was exciting and rewarding. There was a strong bond within the cohort of students at St Thomas's where I secured a place with the offer of three Cs at A level. There are no personal statements in my application in those days, however, my achievements of becoming Deputy Head Boy, Villiers House Captain, Assistant Sea Scout Leader and attainment of the gold Duke of Edinburgh Award helped me stand out from the others. In the long summer vacations, I was fearless and confident and, using the salesman skills I learned as a relief milkman and absorbed from listening to my father, I convinced the panel to give me a place. These attributes were to stand me in good stead but also led to me being almost crushed by 'the organisation', our NHS, not once but three times in my 45-year medical career.

Medical training began with two preclinical years including by today's standards a small cohort of 60 medical students at St Thomas' Hospital.

I dissected cadavers to learn human anatomy, carried out experiments on fellow students in physiology and tried to make organic chemistry practical experiments work. In the dissection room our group of six had a 'swear box' I introduced, as there was much frustration for novice anatomy students armed with scalpels, forceps and greasy fingers attempting to identify the sural nerve or an adductor femoral artery branch buried in fat and connective tissue. We got used to the smell of formalin after a few sessions. I was the only one who did not contribute pennies to the swear box! Physiology, however, was my forte and I enrolled in the intercalated BSc course. One unit of study was cardiovascular and respiratory, another the nervous system. We experimented on anaesthetised animals in first-floor lab of the Sherrington School of Physiology (animals residing in the animal house on the top floor) and successfully reproduced first-hand, some seminal discoveries important to modern-day medical practice.

Without my realising the impact, I became a local celebrity in a famous experiment on carotid body reflexes when a novel electrode was in my preparation. It was one of those incidents that by chance led to a new discovery. I left a three-way tap turned the wrong way and as it was connected to an artery, the animal was haemorrhaging blood. A manometer was recording blood pressure and as this fell the potassium electrode recorded a dramatic rise in concentration of this ion in the blood. A research fellow, with FRCS, studying for an MS thesis was investigating this recently invented probe and realised what had happened, but this finding of the effect of haemorrhage on potassium, although acknowledged in his thesis, was not published in the scientific papers that followed in the Journals. A series of experiments was subsequently planned 'to investigate this phenomenon'. The research fellow and an author of these papers was to become an internationally renowned cardiothoracic surgeon.

Following this unit of study an opportunity arose to do a project in the Department of Aviation Medicine in Farnborough. I was investigating the role of neck movements on the ocular reflex as part of research into the Air Force's interest in designing head-mounted sights for fighter pilots. This involved recruiting unsuspecting candidates or air cadets, to undergo 'sine-wave' oscillations of the head on the body at varying frequencies. The deal was simple. I strapped them into a swivel chair with their head fixed into a frame above so that it did not rotate with the chair. Electrodes stuck onto the skin near the eyes recorded eye movements and my responsibility was to swing the chair from left to right through 90° in time to a metronome set at varying frequencies to achieve sine-wave movements, so stimulating the nerves in the neck! There was a 'stop' to be sure there was no excessive rotation of their head on their torso! With a clever mathematician and computer graphics we plotted the results on the paper dot printer (no clever software-drawing programmes in 1977) for analysis. Scientific papers followed with my name as an author, my first publication in a medical journal[7]. The final assessment of my BSc included this coursework and a three-hour exam and I was rewarded for my efforts with First Class Honours in Physiology.

The following three years of clinical training consisted of attachments to a series of 'firms' where students in short white coats, pockets stuffed with books on 'how to' and attired with stethoscope and patella hammer, followed the Houseman, SHO, Registrar, Senior Registrar and Consultant on 'safari' ward rounds. Having spent three years sitting on wooden benches in lecture theatres our feet ached by mid-morning, and we wondered how these 'real' doctors managed to stay on their feet all day! Gradually gaining confidence as we grew into the potential doctors of the future NHS, we had drummed into us the privileged role in society we were soon to attain was dependent on our integrity and professionalism, maintaining standards, not wavering from the moral and ethical teaching we had repeatedly imprinted onto our cortex. This was truly a 'higher calling'. We were expected to uphold this throughout our careers.

My social life as a St Thomas's medical student was relatively benign by standards of the time, with regular 'Hops' at St Thomas's House and a bar serving free-flowing Young's beer. The Christmas shows were the highlight of the year with multitalented medical students performing on stage and letting their hair down. Famously the 'Instant Sunshine' trio (genitourinary consultants) played the show out with cleverly written musical sketches. Instant Sunshine is three dinner-jacketed men of a certain age, singing their original humorous songs, gently mocking the British way of life.

The three founder members – Peter Christie, David Barlow and Alan Maryon Davis – are still going strong after more than 40 years. Peter who pens the music and lyrics, also plays the guitar, trumpet and ukulele. David is the lead guitarist and doubles on mouth organ and spoons. Alan is the group's percussionist and rubber face. Including the occasional double-bass player Tom Barlow (and his predecessor the late Miles Kington) have wowed audiences as far afield as New York, Hong Kong, New Zealand and Bermuda.

Instant Sunshine has over 100 songs on vinyl, cassette or CD, and have written and performed many signature tunes for radio and TV, including *One-upmanship*, *One is Fun*, *Money Box* and for our own three series of *Jackanory*. In the mid-1980s there were three series of *Instant Sunshine Reasonably Together Again* on BBC Radio 4 (in 1985, 1986 and 1988) which are still occasionally repeated on BBC 7 (renamed BBC Radio 4 Extra April 2011). They had a long association with Radio 4's *Stop the Week* (1975-1992) with a three-minute slot most weeks to sing a song about whatever topic was under discussion – anything from unrequited love to weeding the herbaceous border. In addition, Instant Sunshine has performed privately for the Royal Family and publicly at the North Peckham Civic Centre.

On one occasion the antics of a group of senior students got rather out of hand and a milk churn full of sand, used as a doorstop, mysteriously dropped from the third floor to the bottom stairwell leaving a circular depression a few inches deep on the flagstone floor below. The 'Barnes Wallace Memorial Fund' was formed and it raised enough to repair the damage and a future consultant chest physician had done his penance. So was the nature of medical student life at St Thomas's in the 1970s.

In the third year there was an 'elective' to look forward to, usually six weeks abroad to gain experience in another country. However, many used it as a creative way of a summer holiday. In my case I had two electives, but both were academic and clinical with a short period of travel in their respective continents.

My first excursion was in the second preclinical year during obstetrics when I and another student in my firm Oenone Brown (married, now Warr), devised a research project and secured ethical approval and sponsorship to pay for us to travel to India. In India, the 'caste system' is perpetuated today. Many mothers we saw came from lower casts in poor health and were undernourished. Ethical clearance was necessary and formal consent integral to the methodology, obtained with translation from local staff. The aim was to measure blood glucose levels in malnourished mothers and look for any correlation with birth weight of their baby. We travelled to the Punjab and recruited mothers and babies, keeping their placentas and taking blood samples, making measurements in all of these. The most entertaining challenge was sending these blood samples home to St Thomas's. It is important to realise in the days when we were students, things were different. There was little problem bringing flasks of liquid nitrogen from the biochemistry lab to freeze blood samples to -70°C, pack them in dry ice in a cool-box and then transport them by second-class train to Delhi and then onto a plane for a courier and to be collected at Heathrow Airport by our professor of endocrinology. On arrival at St Thomas's our professor took the prized cargo to the pathology department where they underwent HbAlc measurements, a novel diabetic marker of chronic blood glucose levels. Another publication followed, with us as two medical students as first authors[9].

Oenone Warr

Hello Lance,

I have found an old photograph album and a copy of the paper we produced. It seems such a long time ago. Already you and your wife had found each other so there is a nice photo of you both.

I remember that organising the logistics of the finance was complex. We were struggling to justify going to India rather than an English Hospital; the scientific theory came together, and the project evolved under the expert ideas of Maureen Young in Obstetrics and Professor Bill Cranston, head of the medical unit. (Professor Bill Cranston and Professor Young have passed away since). Professor John Anderson also supported us financially with a grant from a hospital fund. It was fun, but hard work and culturally very challenging. We are very privileged. We worked extremely hard. We had extraordinary train rides transporting frozen blood samples from Ludhiana to St Thomas's. Jane Tavinor, a physio also came with us. It was the most extraordinary achievement.

My memories are you were always hard working and logical. I don't remember you ever losing your temper or being anything apart from focused and involved in the science. It was fascinating to work in such a distant hospital with the extraordinary train journeys to deliver blood samples to the airport to fly back to St Thomas's London for The HbA1C levels etc.

We met amazing doctors and many kind people who helped us including the charming Indian family in Delhi the Vermas. Through them we were able to experience a home in Delhi, join a vintage car race and celebrate the engagement of their daughter Wanita. At that party I met Gita Menon who is now a consultant anaesthetist in London and a close friend.

Oenone

Jane Tavinor found her experience a life changing one. Here are her memories.

A Crossroads in Life

In the late 1970s, I was at a crossroads in life. Fresh out of school and physiotherapy training, I felt the pull to see more of the world beyond my comfortable childhood. India called to me, offering a baptism of fire to the vast, vibrant world beyond the confines of my teenage years. I flew to Ludhiana on my own, ready to throw myself into a research project at the Christian Medical College Hospital, a venture organized by two of my sister's friends from medical school: Lance and Oenone.

The adventure began the moment I stepped off the plane. Delhi airport felt like pure madness, an exhilarating chaos that left me wide-eyed and buzzing with a mix of excitement and nerves. Navigating the complexities of Indian railways, figuring out ticketing systems, and even simple things like haggling with vendors were challenges I'd never faced. But those early moments of confusion were just the beginning of my immersion into a world so different from anything I'd known.

With a tingle of anticipation, I managed to catch the right train to Ludhiana, experiencing the sights and sounds of India from the train window—steam locomotives chugging past, chai wallahs weaving through the carriages, and peanut sellers making their rounds. The pulse of the country was everywhere, and I was both overwhelmed and thrilled by it all.

Once I arrived at the Christian Medical College I met Lance and Oenone. We got along from the outset. Oenone and I forming an allegiance early to counter whenever Lances drive and energy exceeded ours!! The work on the project began. Lance took charge of the planning, a natural leader with a determination that drove the project forward, even when others might have faltered. Oenone and I, though not exactly shrinking violets, often disagreed on how best to proceed. But those debates, while challenging at times, pushed us to think more creatively I felt. Despite those tensions we formed a team, and the work was balanced by the joy of our shared humour and the unforgettable experiences we had along the way.

The hospital, a microcosm of India's warmth and hospitality, became our home. We met doctors and staff who treated us like family, and soon we were traveling to nearby towns and villages, invited to weddings, vintage car rallies, and the annual staff picnic. I particularly remember the elderly English doctors who had spent decades working in India, their expertise and compassion shaping the local medical landscape, particularly in treating deformities caused by leprosy in rural communities.

Lance, with Oenone's support, orchestrated impossible feats. There was the night train to Delhi with frozen blood samples in hand, heading to the airport to be sent back to London. We spent the journey curled up on the train floor, clutching the box of blood samples There was something magical about these late-night train rides, sharing a small piece of the country's vastness with people who had become dear to me. When we arrived in Delhi, we were welcomed by Oenone's family friends, the wonderful Vermas, who offered us comfort, kindness, and a sense of belonging. This gave me the freedom to explore Delhi, where I wandered through the streets, absorbing the sights, sounds, and smells of a place that had started to become familiar to me.

The research itself was sometimes tedious work. My small room in a leafy courtyard was where we gathered to plan, while I meticulously extracted triglycerides from blood samples. Lance would chase down placenta samples like Dracula after blood, keeping me occupied with his energetic, all-consuming drive. He could organize anything—liquid nitrogen, vacuum flasks, you name it—there was no problem too big for him to solve.

In between the hours of lab work, we took tea breaks in the hospital courtyard canteen, where the chai wallah served the most delicious, sweet, hot tea and we shared life stories and made plans for our travels.

The living arrangements were simple: a barn-like building with cubicles, and an outdoor bathroom heated by a wood-fired boiler. The hot water was a luxury, but the laughter and camaraderie more than made up for any discomfort. The small, intimate struggles of daily life became a backdrop to the larger, more fulfilling moments of the trip.

After the project was finished, our paths diverged and converged once again. I took a long, scenic train ride down to the south of India while Lance and Oenone flew. We met up in Kerala, exploring temples and getting fully immersed in the vibrant life of the country. But eventually, we parted ways. They flew back home, and I continued on for another few months, each of us carrying a piece of India with us.

Reflecting back on that month, I hold the memories of my time with Lance and Oenone close to my heart. Lance, the dynamic driving force of the team, and Oenone, his ever-willing partner in crime, made the impossible possible. They were an unstoppable duo. I wrote to my family that I had full confidence in Lance to achieve anything—somehow, he would always find a way to make it happen. Though he still managed to get the flight times to Patna wrong……!!!

Those months in India, guided and enriched first by my time with Lance and Oenone, shaped and changed my life. It was a time of growth, of learning to navigate the complexities of research, travel, and relationships, all set against the backdrop of one of the most fascinating places on earth. It opened my eyes to the world. It changed my life.

What an amazing time that was

Jane x

My other project as a preclinical medical student on the medical unit firm involved aspirating saliva from the salivary duct inside the cheeks of diabetic patients attending clinics and measuring glucose concentrations and blood glucose levels simultaneously. Another publication from St Thomas's students followed[10].

In my final year I also took my elective abroad, this time I travelled to Malawi and gained experience in tropical medicine in a small missionary hospital. The obstetric service was run single-handed by a consultant who taught me how to do a caesarean section using conscious sedation, local anaesthetic and one catgut suture to repair the uterus after delivery of the newborn. Materials were scarce and nothing went to waste. This experience of feeling I made a real difference to the lives of these wonderful patients who existed in conditions of poverty unimaginable until seen firsthand is never lost on me.

I travelled the length of Malawi hitchhiking, walking through small villages of mud dwellings, and exchanging a bag of salt for a bed for the night and to buy a memento. A wooden carving of a man smoking a pipe was a prize find. I named him 'Banda' after the president and he resides in my bedroom in our home today. The final year came to an end as all our minds were focused on passing our exams to become qualified doctors. The oral exams (vivas) brought many to a quaking mess and the written exams covered such a wide curriculum that much cramming of facts occurred late into the long nights of pre-exam panic. Yet despite all the stress, most of us passed first time, soon to brave the wards as junior doctors.

My recollection of the day after the results was waking up in a first-class railway carriage, having slept past my station with three pints of Young's best beer slowly metabolising. Too slowly, for my liver was used to only half a pint! The train guard found me in the second-class carriage as we pulled into the station with the last train of the night and my explanation that I had just graduated as a doctor must have been the clincher, as he let me into the adjoining first-class carriage, put on the heaters and as he left the car he wished me good luck and a safe return home the next day, a true gesture of kindness.

I was on top of the world. My ambition of being a doctor was now a reality.

Chapter 3

Early Impressions 1978

As a medical student starting on the wards, it was an exciting and daunting experience. The long days trekking around the wards on safari ward rounds were soon part of my routine and I could concentrate on learning the skills of taking history from the patient and performing examinations. It soon became clear to me each of us was struggling to do what seemed so easy when observing the registrars in action. Registrar ward rounds were twice daily, and the houseman never left the ward, always reading off telephone extensions flashing up on a bleep while negotiating their endless list of jobs. Some registrars had duties off the wards, outpatient clinics, procedure lists, operating lists, presentations, teaching sessions and departmental meetings, mostly a mystery to us.

The consultant ward round occurred twice a week and never on the weekend. The senior registrar effectively ran the show. On the occasion we joined the consultant ward round, it was an opportunity to hear words of wisdom that came from decades of experience. Consultants were wearing pristine starched long white coats and stood out from the wrinkled more grubby looking now off-white junior doctors' coats. Teaching occurred on these ward rounds and students shuffled their places hoping to avoid being the first one to take a history and examine a patient. In my case I would more often than not volunteer first, prepared to get it wrong knowing I would learn and retain more from earlier mistakes rather than watching passively an A-grade student doing the perfect examination and reeling off the textbook diagnosis. There were a few who had encyclopaedic knowledge and photographic memories. I had to constantly apply myself by overcoming the fear of making a mistake and it soon became clear most of my peers were happy to let me take the pressure off them. We supported each other and a strong bond was rapidly formed between us.

The one highlight of the day was attending the lunchtime post-mortems where the pathologist would hold court like a gladiator in a Greek arena. The cadaver had already been dissected and the organs displayed on a large bench-top surrounding the mortuary. Weighing scales and measuring jugs stood expectantly until they were individually brought into action by the assistant, at the command of the 'conductor', our professor of pathology.

Medical students would be standing three or four rows deep looking down at the scene. The demonstration would begin with a summary of the case and how the patient ended up on the cold slab for the post-mortem. The pathologist would scan the lines of students, seeing the nervous expressions and eyes turning away to avoid contact in case the first question of the day came their way. It was a nervous moment as the poor student who landed with the first question; "Now, sonny. What is the organ I am holding up?" He raised a large purple saggy object, dripping brown fluid onto the table and continued. "And what is the pathology?", the student now turning crimson and aware of his contemporaries silently waiting and knowing how the scene played out. He made his best guess at the abomination held aloft. "Err … A liver, sir. … I … I think it's probably cirrhotic?" Then the put-down, the humour the laughter, the smiles, the wink and the nod from the professor of pathology as he replied, "Good guess, my son. This is a set of lungs. …' Laughter, and everyone waits for the killer punch, " … full of water. Did you not see the stuff dripping out?" He squeezes the lungs gently to demonstrate efficiently how wet they are. "This patient died of heart failure, and this is what pulmonary oedema is."

The student replied in a quiet voice, "That was my alternative thought," to more laughter. The game was on and the professor came out with his famous phrase, "Let this lesson be written in tablets of stone upon your heart so you will never forget." We never forgot. There was a fantastic way of learning and real entertainment at the same time.

Now we all realised the privileged position we were in as these were our patients who had recently been on our ward or admitted B.I.D (brought in a dead) and there was immense respect shown by his careful handling and placement of the body parts as the verbal exchanges played out. His body language made it quite clear that this was a serious demonstration. We were in awe of the extensive knowledge of the pathologist, and all appreciated the humour as a means of minimising the inevitable stress all of us seeing recently dead bodies, dissected organs weighed, measured, sliced to show their interior structures then counted and placed in order on the benches in front of us. We had all dissected cadavers in our anatomy class, but this was not the same. We learned how fragile life is and how death is only seconds away. Then we had our lunch and returned to the wards to see our patients.

It required practice to compartmentalise these experiences and emotions. Respect for a consultant grew with his or her experience and we knew we had a long way to go before becoming a doctor. About ten percent of the original student cohort would leave medicine for other careers when they realised this was not their calling.

I recall one ward round when attached to the professor of medicine firm (Bill Cranston, believe it or not, he was a smoker in those days) and the senior registrar brought our group to the bedside of the patient and asked me to look at the fundi (back of the eye) using an ophthalmoscope. Now this is a difficult skill to master (and nowadays has not been taught to many students properly) as first you must learn how to work the instrument. There are varying types, and you need to check if the batteries are flat or if you have not turned it on, whether it is a plug-in version. Then, is the room dark enough? If not, the pupils are going to be too small without eye drops. If that is the case, there is no chance of seeing the retina at the back of the eye.

Next you have to locate the blood vessels and trace them towards the central disc and orientate yourself. In doing this it is easy to head-butt the patient unless you place a hand on their forehead. I took the ophthalmoscope and the light worked, the beam was the large white one, so my next task was to find the red spot shining the light at the pupil from a few centimetres away then move to within a centimetre or two from the cornea. I found the disk, the blood vessels thinning out in a star formation, one at 2 o'clock, another 10 o'clock, the third at 5 o'clock and the last back at 7 o'clock. I altered the angle of the beam to trace the course of each artery in turn along its course towards the perimeter of the retina. What I saw I had not read about or seen in my houseman's pocket 'how-to-do' book and wished I had access to the large *Atlas of Ophthalmology* sitting on the shelf in the library. I am sure I walked past this on several occasions. Too late, I reverted to the strategy we were taught to pass our 'viva'; describe what you see, explain what it could be then make an educated guess at the diagnosis.

The senior registrar picked me because he knew I was enthusiastic and most eager to impress when in a group. Although I was clearly not the cleverest, I had no photographic memory to draw on, not being one for reading large textbooks, but relied on my notetaking and lectures and seeing as many patients as I could. None of this helped now. My senior registrar then spoke a phrase I will never forget; "Dr Forbat," (yes he addressed me as if I was one) "now is the time to show us your mettle." I didn't recall hearing this term before but knew I was under the spotlight and had to rise to the challenge. 1 described several pale circular areas around the outer rim of the optic nerve, close but not encroaching on it. Each white disk had a very fine black rim. I paused, took a breath, guessed or retrieved a memory from somewhere hidden in my cortex and blurted out my answer. "Laser burns." I looked around at my colleagues waiting for a reaction and then the follow-up question "And why might that be?" I remember seeing the patient receiving injections one ward round and my second guess was more informed. "He is a diabetic." "Correct. So why are we burning his eyes when his vision is poor?" "New vessels are growing over the light-sensitive cells in his retina his treatment killed off those, so they could not proliferate anymore." This was teaching at his best, encouraging students to think on his or her feet. Making them feel out of their comfort zone and see how they cope. This is the experience required to be a good doctor, as we will be put in this situation every day of our careers. It served to reinforce this knowledge so that to this day 47 years later I still see myself in a short grubby off-white coat, standing over this patient and trying "to find my mettle". On that day I struck gold. To me today this answer was obvious.

Many times since I have relived the scene and still use it in my teaching sessions. Those students who stood watching me I have no doubt gained new knowledge by observing a fellow student being politely grilled by the senior registrar.

This was an example of the best of medical education and replicated many times in my student years. These were my first impressions of what a good doctor was all about.

Then day came with the realisation that not every doctor held the same standards. Overhearing a conversation in the corridor as I came out of the lift, I witnessed a senior transplant surgeon "squaring up" to the senior physician, his face contorted in a rage while the opposition stood in serene calmness in his pristine starched white coat. I did not catch the whole exchange from the beginning, but it was clear they were at odds over the dose of diuretic to give a transplant patient. This was the first of many such confrontations I saw between consultant colleagues, surgeons, and physicians and surgeons versus other surgeons. It was an eye-opener. This was my second impression of early years in medicine. There was a glimpse of Bobby Manson confronted by Chibbs Telford of SAMCRO. Then there was the confrontation between a senior cardiothoracic surgeon throwing a tantrum (possibly Lee Toric) towards the quietly standing figure of another eminent senior cardiologist (exhibiting the characteristics of Cons, the honest policeman). Bubbling up from under the surface, I saw in my future medical colleagues the same personality traits exhibited by characters in the *Sons of Anarchy*, albeit diluted in real life. However, as a mere medical student, I only saw the tip of the iceberg. I had to wait until I was a qualified doctor in the real world and working 'cheek by jowl' with my consultant colleagues, before witnessing how the expression of primordial drivers of the complex human condition was not restricted to a criminal motorbike gang. *(Page 190 Scene – A tense meeting between Toric and Chibs, and Scene – "The Clubhouse")*

Chapter 4

An Education and More 1980

Now I was a doctor, a pre-registration house physician on a one-in-two on-call rota. That meant working 24 hours every other day and weekends. The weekend on-call starts at nine in the morning on Friday and ends at five in the afternoon on Monday and the next on-call night is Tuesday and then on Thursday following this. This amounts to 120 hours a week on duty. Pay was at one-third hourly rate after the first 40 hours, or ten UMTs (Units of Medical Time) so long hours were essential to get a mortgage. In these first six months I was on the renal unit firm, and my responsibility was to manage very sick patients on dialysis and undergoing renal transplantation. None had decent veins to take blood or to insert a drip line. It was a steep learning curve. The senior registrars were older than today's newly qualified consultants, with extensive experience as they marked time waiting for a consultant to retire or die, in order to release a vacancy for promotion.

During the next six months I was a surgical houseman in Canterbury and had fought hard to secure a particular placement as I had a taster in my student attachment here. It was my most memorable, assisting in emergency surgery in a variety of cases and learning to suture with the dexterity of a surgeon. I removed an appendix, assisted in repairing an inguinal hernia and assisted in other cases under the supervision of the senior surgical registrar. As a house surgeon I was given increasing responsibility. I was expected to have formulated a plan for all my patients, up to 30 on any day. "What is the plan?", my consultant would ask for each patient at the bedside. This firm worked a one in two-week on-call system. There was also Sunday clerking for the patients admitted for assessment by the anaesthetist 'gassing' at the Monday morning list, even when not on call. This meant I was continuously available for emergency admissions from 9am on Monday morning until the next Monday afternoon at 5pm and every Sunday morning clerking regardless of not being on duty. Also, there was no phlebotomist for blood-taking after mid-morning weekdays and none on weekends. All fell to me.

My realisation was much of what we learned at medical school did not prepare me for the duties of the Houseman. Most seemed redundant to the daily chores of form filling, bloodletting, putting in drip lines and ringing the GP after every death on our surgical firm, an expectation of our consultant of 'the old school'.

I was married soon after qualifying and my wife, by then a qualified nurse, followed me from London to Canterbury, sharing the sleep deprivation as a consequence of a one-in-two rota. Yet despite all this lack of sleep, fatigue and little social life, we felt valued as part of the family working toward a common goal, giving our all to care for our patients. This was the NHS I grew up with. This was the 'more' required of the doctor that a formal medical student education could not provide. Led by example, see one, learn one, do one, was the apprenticeship we lived and worked. Exposure to sick and injured patients daily was littered with traumatic facial injuries arriving in casualty due to car crashes on the A2 in the pre-seatbelt era. Surgery on the head and neck (maxillofacial surgery) was in daily demand.

One night I was on call with a locum surgical registrar when a man was admitted after his wife plunged a breadknife into his abdomen during a domestic row. He had a tachycardia (rapid heart rate) overnight and the registrar decided just to observe him. On the morning consultant ward round my presentation of the case was a lesson I will never forget. The patient was still unwell and had a low blood pressure despite a transfusion. My consultant took one look at the man and said, "Theatre. Now." In the space of 10 minutes or so he was on the table, and my consultant was wielding a scalpel. He opened his chest with a swift cut to the side of the sternum to expose the heart and blood oozing from a tear in the pericardium where the bread knife had risen up from its entry point in the abdomen through the diaphragm to the chest close to the heart. With one stitch the leak was sealed, the heart rate settled and he closed the chest. There was no cardiac surgeon on this site, but my consultant was a general surgeon who had seen action in the field of battle. This was not the only lesson to a young Houseman two months into his surgical experience. On leaving the accident and emergency ward to go to the operating theatre, my consultant turned to me and raising his voice said, "You're MY houseman! You should've called me immediately. This patient could have died!" I replied, "I said it was the registrar in charge who decided to observe him overnight." That did not wash. "You are MY houseman and I expect you to inform me about all sick patients, day or night."

Every weekend on-call and Sunday clerking I dutifully rang my consultant at home (no mobiles in those days) and relayed the progress of each and every new patient giving my plan for each as expected. This was true delegation of responsibility and certainly character-building. We were a team, a family and there was trust. Ward rounds always broke for tea and biscuits in sister's office. Also, my wife and I were invited for Sunday lunch at his home with his family. That was the NHS in this era, in this hospital and this consultant. It was not the experience of all newly qualified doctors and since then the NHS has become unrecognisable. The phrase "in my day" had a real meaning behind it and still influences the way I take my responsibilities today.

The notion of continuous education I called "the more" in my experience, cannot be overemphasised. Following guidelines and online learning, lectures by eminent professors and walking the walk are not the same. Ticking boxes is not caring and turning a blind eye to omissions and mistakes does the profession and patients no favours. Experience counts and respect gains respect.

I was now ready to make a career decision. I had my taste of surgery, so intense on a job I fought for because I knew I wanted to be a physician and I knew this time spent would satisfy my desire to explore the "other side". The division is stark and yet neither can function without the other and understanding both is the central for the rounded physician. Knowing when to refer, when to ask for help and most importantly to trust your judgment.

Throughout my period as a medical student and my pre-registration year as a houseman, I was becoming more aware, how the human factors shaping our world; ambition, jealousy, greed, narcissism, bullying, scheming, power struggles, politics, crime, sex also determine the nature of the NHS. These attributes transcend society's barriers and as I was watching I saw all these attributes played out by the characters in the setting of a criminal motorbike gang of the SAMCRO charter (c.f the firm) in the town of Charming and all at war with the rival firms or Charters, including the Mayhan, China's, Stockholm Charters and many more.

My early impressions were formed and reinforced as I progressed up the medical career ladder. These did not shake my belief in doing the right thing, speaking up when circumstances arose, that turning the other cheek was not an option for me. In the next few chapters, I reveal how human nature in all its guises has shaped the once admirable vision of Nye (Aneurin) Bevan's NHS and has been usurped by those I call "The Sons of Bevan".

So, you may be wondering what similarity is there to *Sons of Anarchy*? (Episode 1, "The Pilot", see page 189). Some of the main characters in *Sons of Anarchy* are given their likely roles in the NHS as *avatars* but not necessarily gender specific to their roles here. I have only named those involved where in the public domain, but each will have to search their conscience, as they will know exactly which role they played.

Chapter 5

The Real World 1981

In my introduction, I set the scene with a brief overview of my first substantive consultant post and a most recent locum appointment. To reach consultant status in the 1990s required 10 to 15 years of short-term contracts, moving regularly and passing exams to progress through the system. Having gained first class BSc honours it helped for the first year or so, but without passing part one and part two of membership for Royal College of Physicians, it was not possible to progress to registrar grade. Working in SHO posts in neurology, cardiology and respiratory firms on onerous rotas of one-in-two and one-in-three on call did not leave much time for study and it took me three attempts to pass my part one membership and after a two-year interlude I passed my part two, opening the door to a registrar post. I secured a two-year rotation in gastroenterology and renal medicine and had not yet decided on my professional specialty to follow until later than most. The attraction of cardiology was closely associated with my interest in physiology. However, I was initially put off the speciality earlier in my time as a medical student at St Thomas's by the infighting I observed between the Cardiac Surgeons and Cardiology consultants. I could not envisage life with so much discord going forward. Over time however and following my SHO cardiology post, I realised it was the individuals more than the specialty at the root of the problems. The competitiveness of ascending the specialist ladder to consultant status attracted certain types of personality and once the status of consultant was reached (e.g , personalities that were suppressed in order to secure suitable references and navigate the appointment panels were now unchecked for the first time. Politics became a large part of the consultant's brief as management decisions, finance and other pressures of competing departments came into play.

My first SHO post was in a private wing of a hospital as I was studying for membership, and this meant looking after a whole mix of medical and surgical patients. The job was coordinating the daily management of private patients and dealing directly with consultants. There was no intermediate registrar or senior registrar between the consultant and me. It was soon apparent how private practice affected individual consultants' attitudes toward me as a junior in different ways. Some are warm, polite and encouraging, others brash, authoritarian and often insufferable and yet the patients adored them and trusted them implicitly.

I learned more about bedside manner and how to bring or break bad news to patients in the six months by listening firsthand to the interaction between consultant and patient than any teaching sessions. Humour was a major part of many encounters. I vividly recall a cardiac surgeon seeing his patient after returning from ITU to the private wing following open-heart surgery. The patient was in his sixties and had been looking at his healing sternotomy wound, when the surgeon came in to inspect his progress. He had a large tattoo on his chest, and he complimented the consultant on lining up the pattern of his tattoo so perfectly. The consultant looked at the results closely and said, "Well, I opened your chest and did my operation and then thought, that will do. I will chuck it all back in and it will fit somehow. As long as I make a neat scar at the end, you won't know any different!" He knew his patient better than I, as the patient let out a huge laugh and had to hold his chest to stop it moving too much. He is one of the neatest surgeons I've seen operate and even invented a tissue valve. During any spare time, he was a keen sailor and often compared yachts and argued about who owned the best fast car with his other well-heeled consultant colleagues. Another consultant was a prima donna and dressed like a pop star with open neck shirt, gold medallion necklace on show (images of Chuck Marston). However, I was not party to how these consultants were perceived in their roles within the NHS system. I remembered the privileged role in society we held was dependent on our integrity and professionalism, maintaining standards, not wavering from the moral and ethical teaching that we were expected to uphold throughout our careers.

My next SHO post was in cardiology in an old TB hospital the Brook, that was soon to close, where I had my first real taste of cardiology. I experienced another delightful team comprising a Consultant Dr Max Zoob and Associate Specialist Dr Stacky Guertner, reinforcing my interest in cardiology. In the nine months here I passed my part one membership so preparing the way to a registrar appointment following this post. I had an SHO job back at St Thomas's in the neurology department. This was based on Florence ward, so I was already known to the staff and where previously as a medical student and (on Independence Day 4th of July 1978!) with my friend David Jones looking for nurses to attend the orthopaedic/psychiatric firm party, I invited a very efficient ward receptionist, now my wife. I asked David recently if he could recall the orthopaedic/psychiatric firm party at St Thomas's when I asked the ward receptionist on Florence to join us. "I can't remember much about your wife, only that I remember seeing her on the ward and how smitten you were!!" What I recall of David is we had the same zany sense of humour, or at least he put up with mine! He was a keen hockey player and on the one occasion he broke a leg and it was in plaster, I sent him one of my cartoons of him in a wheelchair with plastered leg extended while hurtling at speed, hair flowing in the wind, as I imagined he might along the tiled corridors of St Thomas's. Ward rounds included a gaggle of students and junior doctors following their consultant, changing floors using a paternoster lift, a passenger elevator which consists of a chain of open compartments (each usually designed for two people) that move slowly in a loop up and down inside a building without stopping. We were all hoping to see one miss a step or crowding in three or four to a cubicle. It was like a large bicycle chain and at the top went round and came down the other side with new passengers. I decided this was not enough excitement for the new students on initiation to St Thomas's, so I demonstrated how to time the stepping on and off and with practice, jumping as late as one dared. Up I went and out of sight to the novices. As I reached the top of the ride, I did a handstand and came down the other side on my head. I think it had the desired effect! David sent his recollections, unaware of my memories above and we concurred on many and he added many I had forgotten!

For your memoirs Lance

> *"Those years at St Thomas's between 1977 and 1980 were a rich blend of clinical education, mild chaos, and unfiltered hilarity—and Lance was frequently at the heart of it.*
>
> *I vividly remember one of those particularly long (and, dare I say, soporific) lectures when Lance—armed with nothing but a biro and a mischievous look in his eye—sketched a cartoon of me in a wheelchair, leg in plaster, hooked up to machines by a tangle of tubes and drips. The exact backstory behind my imagined injuries is long forgotten, but we had just finished a firm in orthopaedics and still had colorectal surgery and ENT fresh in our minds from previous firms. I recall we were filled with amazement—tinged with schoolboy humour—at the near-magical capabilities and limitless reach of modern endoscopy. The cartoon may as well have been captioned, "Too much probing, not enough caution!"*

Then there was the unforgettable orthopaedic/psychiatric firm party—a heady mix of bone-setting and mind-bending madness (the firm, not the party!) — where Lance first met the lovely ward receptionist from Florence Ward, his future wife. Who'd have thought that a firm party would spark a marriage? But didn't stop there. His future wife's good friend, the charming nurse Teresa Parsons, caught my eye, and as fate would have it, we too tied the knot in 1983. Lance, never missing a comic beat, marked our wedding day by placing a massive worm—yes, a real one—on the path just as the wedding photos were being taken. Nothing like a squirming prop to keep things memorable.

Ward rounds were rarely dull when Lance was around. There was the paternoster in North Wing—a glorified death trap disguised as a lift. We were warned never to ride it "over the top" for reasons that were never explained… so of course Lance had to do it. He disappeared up and out of sight to the gasps of fellow students, only to descend moments later, upside down in a handstand, grinning like a circus act. The man had balance, style, and absolutely no fear.

And then there was our two-week medical attachment at Worthing Hospital in the summer of '79. A glorious blur of sunshine, half-hearted ward rounds, and suspiciously little actual studying but a lot of talk of his wife to be. We both returned with sunburn that suggested more time on the beach than in the hospital, and I'm fairly sure Lance conducted most of the fortnight with his sunglasses on. Still, we looked impressively tanned for two aspiring physicians... if not entirely competent.

My memories of those years are, like an old medical textbook, slightly dog-eared and full of scribbled notes, but they are bathed in laughter and good friendship. The hops, the mischief, the sneaking into Gassiot House past the Rottweiler of a male receptionist (not easy!) and above all, the enduring camaraderie of our year group. Happy days indeed.

David

In my role as SHO to the neurology firm it became apparent after the first few days that the administrative side of the NHS was in some disarray, with large numbers of patients pending admission for investigation recorded in a large exercise book, but there was no system in place to prioritise these patients. It was my job to arrange admissions, and some had been sitting in the admissions book for a considerable period of time, while the more recent entries were being admitted ahead of these. I went down to the 'Cut', a market under the arches of Waterloo and purchased a pegboard and cards. I wrote a card with the details of each patient waiting with their demographics, diagnosis and most importantly the date of placement on the list. The admissions to the ward immediately started arriving in order of priority as assigned by me, so within six weeks all patients had either been admitted or given a date within two weeks of their listing. I demonstrated my management skills and leadership, and this resulted in references from my consultant that helped me secure my next post.

These recent posts were the most enjoyable and the consultants in the firms set examples I hoped to emulate.

After I passed my membership, I secured my registrar rotation, first as registrar in gastroenterology then in renal medicine. My time in gastroenterology at St. Charles' Hospital in Ladbrook Grove was another happy period in my career with Dr Hugh Baron who had a passion for art in hospitals, as he wrote articles in the BMJ 'Beautifying Hospitals'. I was offered a promotion to senior registrar but declined the offer as I had decided my career would be in cardiology. The renal unit was an intense environment with more responsibility for very sick patients on haemodialysis and management of patients with kidney transplants. There was tension within the unit between the physicians and a transplant surgeon and the unit Sisters also were in a clique and consequently I never felt comfortable in their presence, especially when there were confrontations as I had seen before, although at registrar level the full picture would elude me until I reached the consultant grade.

The patients on dialysis waiting for renal transplants were different from those in other specialties at the time forming close bonds with the staff as they underwent haemodialysis three times weekly. The additional experience gave me valuable insight into the future of consultant life in the NHS. This pattern of good and bad units was one I would see repeated throughout my 33 years as a consultant. One patient, a young black African man was on the list for a transplant (there is a higher incidence of hypertension in African populations and subsequent kidney failure) and we formed a strong bond, possibly as a consequence of his confidence in me being essential for intense interventional therapy, but I also wondered because I treated him like everyone else, this was not something he had experienced as he stood out as different, out of his usual environment. I thought nothing different of him than of other patients on the unit however on the day of his discharge Sister informed me he wanted to see me and say thank you. I entered his room and he handed me a large package and insisted I open it with him. Inside was a beautifully crafted, dark blue leather briefcase. He must have seen me using my battered imitation leather one I brought to work and knew this was something special. Indeed, it lasted a decade of daily use before it wore out, and I replaced it with a similar but lesser model!

In the middle years of my training as a registrar, I had more responsibility and was learning how to lead a team, for example, with running cardiac arrest teams. I was also learning the techniques for dealing with patients' relatives after an unsuccessful resuscitation attempt. As is always the case we made mistakes and did our best and learned from them. In my 46 years as a doctor, I have witnessed patients dying when they need not, who were not offered resuscitation and those who should have been left to die naturally and resuscitation correctly not attempted (DNAR) due to co-morbidities.

This is because their multiple medical issues cannot be corrected by chest compression and a defibrillator, artificial ventilation or drug and death is inevitable and natural outcome. People die in hospitals. However, good care is something we all expect and often this falls down when there is poor leadership, lack of staff, or indifference to others whether due to any form of discrimination when there is a bullying culture and when the reputation of individuals in positions of power or the institution responsible for the service loses sight of the 'why' and fails to learn the 'how' of giving healthcare.

My next goal was to obtain a cardiology registrar post to be in the running for promotion in the speciality. I needed to bolster my CV and obtaining an MD was the best option here. I went back to St Thomas's and the Sherrington School of Physiology where I did my BSc. With the help of the lecturers, I applied and successfully obtained a British Heart Foundation Junior Cardiac Fellowship. There was a six-month delay before funding would come through so I decided to take a year abroad and secured a registrar job at King Khalid National Guard Hospital in Jeddah, Saudi Arabia, and see the some of the world with my wife. This would provide some spare money towards the lean period that the grant income available to me (no extra UMTs) could not match and so afford my mortgage repayments.

The experience I gained here was unique in several ways. Firstly, seeing health provision in a different society outside the NHS model, secondly experiencing a new culture and finally an opportunity to circumvent the world with my wife three months pregnant when we left Jeddah. My wife had suffered hyperemesis in the first trimester, so adding some challenges to a round-the-world trip. The King Khalid National Guard Hospital was within an enclosed compound and was home to expatriates from around the world. There were no restrictions to daily life of Westerners other than the prohibition of alcohol. There was mixed bathing at the swimming pools, spacious air-conditioned apartments and no mosque on campus, until shortly before I left. The majority of staff was European or American and only a handful of Saudi consultants. The juniors were a mixture from around the globe and Saudi graduates made up a significant proportion. The plan was to train these up to Western standards of medicine and then gradually they would replace the expats as they ended their contracts. The environment was different from the NHS in many ways although the service was run along similar lines. There were occasions when a local registrar would disappear for "prayers" and everyone knew it was to avoid particular duties he did not fancy and his compatriots would carry on as normal. Work, however (in medicine) was considered as equivalent to prayers. There was no PALS (patient advisory liaison service) service in the ordinary sense and relatives of the royal family, often many times removed from the centre of the family would gain special access to services and if not satisfied would raise a complaint and this would filter down to the medical director to resolve. During the time we were there, Prince Charles and Lady Diana paid a visit, and this was a real fanfare of an event.

I was acting up as a senior registrar attached to the cardiologist. I was able to gain experience in echocardiography as well as do some local research projects. Relationships were generally very good amongst all the staff there and any politics was well above my head. There were no signs of the *Sons of Anarchy* and versions of SAMCRO in King Khalid National Hospital staff, however, it was a different story within the Kingdom of Saudi Arabia. We heard stories of public beheadings in Riyadh, of bodies being dumped outside private hospitals and residential homes, possibly nurses, healthcare assistants or slaves that transgressed a line. Jeddah was relatively relaxed whereas Riyadh was very strict and had religious police out in force. Women were not allowed to go out unless accompanied by their husbands or a male family member and were not allowed to drive. I had bought a second-hand car so we could explore the area and caution was required when taking photographs of buildings as cameras were confiscated and arrests made. There was one occasion on returning from the souk when my wife leaning out of the car window took a picture of a massive petrol station at night with splendid lighting. She took it out of the car window and unfortunately the flash went off as it was night-time and she hadn't realised it was an automatic camera. I spotted a police vehicle in the rear mirror and as were only a couple of miles from the campus, I put my foot to the floor, and we arrived at the guarded entrance in a few minutes. On being challenged by the century at the barrier I used a cliché I never thought I would "It's all right. I am a doctor working here." This seemed to be enough to let us into the safety of the compound as we watched the police car pass us by at the end of the road leading to King Khalid National Guard Hospital. I never knew if it was following us but being caught was not worth the risk! There were other excursions including 'Wadi bashing', taking a 4x4 into the desert and exploring the rugged terrain. I learned to skin dive in the Red Sea after passing my BSAC (British Sub-Aqua Course) training, beginning in the National Guard swimming pool including learning how to remove and replace the mask, retrieving it from the bottom and expelling the water, buddy breathing off one air supply, open sea training and the use of a depth chart. We did some sailing and frequented the carpet and gold Souks. Checkout lanes at the supermarkets included shelves of grapes, sugar and yeast, not sweets and chocolates, all necessary for making 'Jeddah Gin'.

There are leaders and losers in this world and watching the first few episodes of *Sons of Anarchy* I saw the different characters of SAMCRO played out on screen. It reminded me of real-life power struggles I have experienced and been party to within Nye Bevan's beloved NHS. I decided at around the end of the first few episodes I had my own story waiting to be told and it was time to share it.

Chapter 6

Leaders and Losers 1993

(See Episode 2, "Seeds", page 190.)

In bringing to life this narrative to the reader, especially if unfamiliar with the NHS, I challenge you to imagine a parallel universe. Some physicists have proposed that this landscape, if string theory is true, could give rise to a 'multiverse' and whilst there is no consensus within the scientific community regarding their validity or their potential connection, it has generated considerable debate). In this scenario, I imagined individuals exist simultaneously in a different society and organization, but with similar characteristics and parallel roles.

So you if are still wondering, where do the 'Sons of Bevan' feature in this tale of woe, as I imagined while watching *Sons of Anarchy*? It was unnerving as I immediately saw the similarity in the characters and their roles in our NHS as an organisation. A Hospital Trust hospital is effectively a Charter. Who are the leaders here and what is their responsibility? There is a Chairman of the Board, a Chief Executive Officer and a Finance Officer at the top. They appoint people to various positions and assign their roles to enable the smooth day-to-day running of the organisation. The organisation has a primary duty to service its customers, the patients. The means to achieve this relies on limited sources of income out of their control, so hard decisions have to be made. Within the Charter there are individuals who are vocal and others more passive. The person at the top will have the most influence on who takes on these roles. If it were Clay Morrow, what sort of organisation would it be when compared to Piney Winston at the helm? A Clay Morrow in a Charter would do anything to protect his patch, keeping all the gun contracts in Charming and not be bothered about whom he sells them to. In *Sons of Anarchy*, SAMCRO Charter was selling arms to the real IRA. *(See pages 190–1 – The leader of SAMCRO conspiracy)*

In the NHS today the Chief Executive (*Clay Morrow*) sets the agenda, and it is quite evident from the various scandals from the Bristol Baby Scandal, the executives were criticised for not addressing warning signs and for a lack of transparency. An inquiry led to significant changes in practice and oversight. Subsequently, Stafford Hospital became another scandal. The management were all implicated and therefore the CEO and Trust Chair, as well as other trust leaders, were heavily criticised for failing to prioritise patient safety and for ignoring concerns raised by staff and families[11], as detailed in the subsequent 'Freedom to Speak Up' Francis Report[12]. In more recent events in Morecambe Bay, the leadership was criticised for inadequate risk management and oversight, with calls for accountability and reform in the organisation's practices[13]. The Queen Elizabeth Queen Mother Hospital Margate, faced criticism regarding the standard of care, particularly in maternity services. Investigations into incidents of poor care led to scrutiny of management practices and inadequate responses to complaints, prompting further calls for accountability[14] and many more, that the institutions have lost their way. *(Piney Winston and Jacob Hale Jr, "Addressing the crowd", see page 193)*

A locum consultant will have the same responsibility and hence must be given equal respect and authority expected of all consultants, furthermore in order to maintain this, one relies on support from consultant colleagues. Leading by example is essential in maintaining high standards. In particular for trainees, it is essential for them to have good time keeping, follow up ward round plans in a timely manner, monitor key observations on patients, order tests on time and follow up results and not rely on others by leaving it the next shift. Furthermore, introducing practices to a hospital that are routine and welcomed elsewhere will make one stand out when measured against others. Quality improvement projects (QIP) are encouraged, and juniors are expected to organise these as a requirement of training. This inevitably includes extra work and some of it will be outside the normal daily shift and hence is a voluntary commitment. Completed successfully and signed off by their clinical supervisor leads to 'points' on their CV that increase their success in future job applications. However, having signed up for a project when knowing it meant an extra half hour or so a day, it is often disappointing to find the juniors backing out after a week and showed a lack of commitment, a sad reflection of the 'shift' mentality that has developed since the loss of the firm structure. In the situation I found myself, with the imposition of GMC conditions that were meant to be confidential, where only my supervisor, reporting officer and higher management should be aware, my experience was soon to deteriorate to one of mistrust and undermining of my position.

I was supervising a QIP when some of the juniors involved dropped off the project and as it had started and the department expected it to be completed with an audit. I found I was doing a disproportionate amount of the work. During one period one or two junior doctors in a new intake were not following my management plans and needed repeated prompting. I was concerned, so I raised it with my supervisor who also took part in the project. It has been my experience that some underperforming juniors react negatively when approached about their performance, by complaining to their educational supervisor, who then feeds it back to the clinical leads expecting the consultant to treat them differently. Sometimes if they complain to the Deanery they get supported and the authority of the consultant who is responsible for patient care and their supervision can be undermined. This can lead to dysfunctional teams and worse patient care can result. In one particular week I found that a junior had complained when I asked why they did not follow ward round plans and ignored me when asked if a blood transfusion had been given as requested the previous day. He replied, "I was busy," and turned his back on me. I became concerned that the juniors were now (somehow) aware of my GMC conditions, but my colleague assured me all was confidential. This all changed when the lead consultant confronted the junior doctor for this unacceptable behaviour, who made a revealing statement that shocked us; "Everyone knows Dr Forbat is under investigation by the GMC and has conditions. We have looked him up and even ward sister knows." Fortunately, the issue was resolved and the matter was closed. However, I felt my position had been undermined and it was clear I could no longer work under these circumstances and I resigned.

My feelings at the time were bewilderment that my situation could get this bad and furthermore my absolute frustration. The effect on me was to mistrust those around me and raised anxiety on my part, as well as feeling anger that I should be disrespected by junior doctors who were only recently qualified, very inexperienced and acting so unprofessionally. This lack of respect had potential negative effects on patient care, although I did my utmost to make sure this did not occur, also confiding in a trusted colleague.

To whom it may concern

Letter of Recommendation - Dr Lance N. Forbat (GMC: 2647328)

It brings me great joy to provide this reference for my valued colleague, Dr Lance Forbat who I am privileged to have been acquainted with, since his Locum appointment from 15th September 2021 to 14th October 2022 as a Consultant Physician in Acute Medicine at East Kent Hospitals university foundation trust, Margate, Kent.

Dr Forbat's Physician duties entailed sharing a busy 1:7 acute on-call rota to cover the medical intake as well as providing a senior review on the Accident-Emergency Bay as the in-reaching Acute Physician. His rota also included weekly ward rounds and overseeing any acute emergency in our 27 bedded Acute Medical Unit and providing a Physician led Ambulatory Emergency Care service.

In my capacity as a Lead clinician on the acute and emergency floor - I had the opportunity to oversee Lance's clinical performance wherein he did demonstrate reflective practice and a continuous evaluation of learning and self-performance with excellent knowledge of workplace governance. And provided leadership to a multi-disciplinary workforce consisting of Physicians, junior doctors, critical outreach Nurses and operational teams to re-introduce the Medical Handover.

He also focused on patient flow, understanding the complexity within management and discharge of patients with Heart failure from the Hospital to the community. And provided us with a great insight into the clinical requirements for managing complex heart failure patients with the development of local care solutions such as his proposed 'Diuretic planner'. His involvement with this quality improvement project led to the purchase of appropriate weighing scales for the Emergency floor.

In his pursuit to drive professionalism, Dr Forbat had undertaken an audit to improvise prescribing standards amongst junior doctors. And working with the Pharmacy and Post Graduate Dept., he discussed the need for a signatory stamp that also includes a GMC number to support good prescribing standards.

Furthermore, Dr Forbat also provided educational support for junior doctors in training and willingly contributed to the departmental educational sessions. His ward rounds have been highly commended by trainees - This clearly describes him as an ideal medical teacher who values the growth of intellect *and perception; with the motivation to teach and the desire to learn with an impartial, unbiased attitude - Building a foundation for active participant-driven learning amongst our trainees.*

Lastly, his professional persona, credibility, honesty, and passion to drive efficiency and transparency has been greatly appreciated by me and all members of my staff – I sincerely hope that this reference finds him in good stead, and I have no hesitation in strongly recommending him for the post of consultant physician in Acute and General medicine / Cardiology as he would be a considerable asset to any healthcare organisation appointing him.

Please do not hesitate to contact me if you require any further information. Yours sincerely,

Dr Sunil Lobo

MBBS, PG Cert. (Internal Med.), MRCP UK (Acute Med.), FRCP
Consultant Physician, Acute Medicine
Clinical Lead, Acute & Ambulatory Care, East Kent Hospitals NHS Foundation Trust Hon. Senior Clinical Lecturer, Kings College London
Acute Med. Specialist training committee member, Kent Surrey & Sussex Deanery
Council Member, London & Southeast Regional Clinical Senate

Extracts from the CQC website

The most recent CQC inspection of QEQM Hospital took place in 2019, and the overall rating given was "Requires Improvement." The CQC found that the hospital provided safe, effective, and caring services, but that there were areas where improvements were needed. The hospital was rated as "Requires Improvement" in the categories of safety, responsiveness, and leadership.

The CQC report highlighted several positive aspects of the care provided by the hospital, including that patients were treated with dignity and respect, that staff were caring and compassionate, and that the hospital had a strong culture of safety and learning. However, the report also identified areas where the hospital could improve, such as reducing the length of time patients wait for treatment, improving the management of medicines, and ensuring that there are enough staff to provide safe and effective care.

Incipient in the management structure are close-knit groups facing inwards to protect their positions, resorting to bullying, secrecy, dishonesty and corruption. Monetary gain is the motivation of some individuals, power important in others and a combination of the two in many. The human fallibilities, just as seen in the 'Charters of the Sons of Anarchy' are replicated within our NHS. In the following chapters I tell my own story (at the time I felt as if I was in my own parallel universe of disbelief in that it was happening to me) and relive the collateral damage I experienced, as did the patients that the NHS was formed to serve. A dysfunctional hospital or department is bad for patient outcomes whereas evidence clearly shows that 'Civility Saves Lives'.

These events are real and painful experiences to share. My story is not unique to my personal journey, but (over the decades) multiply it thousands of times across the NHS and you will get some semblance of scale. There are honest, caring hard-working employees who met 'Mr Mayhem', who has many guises (e.g at employment tribunals, the GMC, the encounter even leading to death by suicide) as a result of dysfunctional 'Charters'. This narrative should serve as one more wake-up call to the public and politicians, as the system and its leaders have failed in their duty to their workforce and our patients on a vast scale.[1,4,6] I will expand on this in Chapter 12, "The End Game – Finding Solutions".

Bringing loyal members around the table is achieved by offering fiscal incentives and in the NHS, there are many ways to do this. Appointment to a managerial role such as Clinical Lead or Medical Director usually comes with a temporary uplift in salary for the period of the appointment. Another, and more attractive to the loyal candidate, is a favourable selection for rewards in our discredited points and previous award system. These awards are voted on usually by a group of loyal members of the Charter and anyone not in the cabal, however good their contribution to the institution will, not get any points. First, they may not even get nominated and even if they are shortlisted, will only get the minimum on the scale. Those with some points already and lower awards decided locally, will be best placed for regional and national recognition and so the system is self-serving. The other way to get extra income is through private practice. However, this is not usually influenced by the Trust, especially if it brings in extra revenue when done on their premises. The allocation of extra waiting list clinics can be directed towards favoured individuals. More subtle instruments are the allocations of office space, secretaries and outpatient clinics, also bargaining chips that could be used. Similarly paid study leave applied for will need approval at the Reaper's Table so, as with any action by the Charter, is always confirmed by the clatter of the gavel on the Reaper's Table, study leave requires the signature of the Medical Director or nominated member.

Finally, the use of more aggressive actions such as disciplinary hearings are easily enforced to put any perceived maverick consultant under pressure to back off. The ultimate weapon is "garden leave" or suspension with loss of practicing privileges in the private sector, as income from here is often relied on for school fees and mortgage payments. The potential outcome of an investigation is dismissal from the Trust and raises fear of loss of future pension contributions.

All these levers are on the side of the Trust and a referral to the GMC, on charges, that have often been found to be false (c.f whistleblowers Dr Steve Bolsin, Dr Raj Mattu[15], Dr Chris Day[16]) leading to Mr Mayhem appearing on the scene and a career can be ended or blighted for years. The dismissal of the whistleblower from the Trust may help to persuade the GMC to remove the 'mantle of fitness to practice' from a doctor so ending their career and removing any threat to the Trust, akin to expulsion of a biker from the Charter, terminating membership by removing the tattoo of the Reaper on the biker's back and giving him the grim choice of cutting it off with a knife or burning it off with a flame torch.

This is the feedback I have received from the from the HCSA on this process; "*It is well understood that a trust may refer a doctor after dismissing them via an unfair MHPS process or SOSR, to the GMC as the 'icing on the cake'. I have been told that they are in fact more likely to refer if you resign before the end of the MHPS process as a threat to make you complete the MHPS (which looks better for the trust). The whole process is known to be unfair – MHPS, SOSR and any GMC referral*".

I have met Mr Mayhem three times in my career leaving permanent scars on my family and me. There is an imbalance of power and Trusts are virtually immune to any sanctions if they get it wrong. The Charter fears the whistleblower, as characterised by Juan Carlos "Juice" Ortiz who rats on SAMCRO to the FBI. The 'rat' will find there is no protection as the damage is done before any realistic chance of defending their case can be mustered. The newly appointed 'Freedom to Speak Up Guardian' is in the pay of the Trust and not truly independent of the charter. Invoking the PIDA law (Public Information Disclosure Act), was designed to protect the whistleblower, but in my opinion and according to many, is essentially toothless in protecting the whistleblower. In the recent ongoing case involving Dr Chris Day it became clear, then 10 years ago, that junior doctors were not protected and the HCSA reiterates the commonly held view that for a doctor, your career is over by the time you get to the courts. So, even if PIDA worked, it is too late unless the culture changed in the workplace as a result of it working.

The culture in the NHS as no doubt envisaged by Nye Bevan, has morphed from an open charitable nature, and has been dismantled and re-modelled by the 'interlopers' or 'Sons of Bevan' into the current mess of politically driven and divided Charters that now form its corporate being. Also, within the Charters, just as Clay and Gemma Kemp, they seek to maintain control. Gemma wasn't above lying or betraying members of the club if it suited her needs.

She concealed important information, fabricated stories, and engaged in schemes that put the club at risk. This deceit often resulted in violent confrontations and disrupted the unity of the club. So, departments and the different members form silos. Doctors, nurses, physiotherapists, technicians, pharmacists, secretaries, receptionists, and porters are served up with what managers deem necessary to maintain the service, initially with honourable intentions. Yet it only takes a Clay Morrow or Gemma Teller to infiltrate the top layers of management and medical staffing to destabilise the system using the well-worked principle of 'divide and rule'. Those in the NHS will be very aware of this but are powerless to influence the culture that is so ingrained. The BMA, HCSA and other unions of the allied medical services will have minimal impact on decision making, usually mopping up the collateral damage after Mr Mayhem has done his work.

Anyone working in the National Health Service might expect Occupational Health Services to give support to staff when they fall ill or are unwell. In my case it was a double-edged sword; the Trust wanted me to attend occupational health for a mental health assessment (page 8 of the HCSA's Playbook). I did not feel this was necessary as I had no mental health issues then, before or since. I was concerned that this assessment could be a reason to discredit and exclude me. Janet Eastham, *The Telegraph* journalist on 15 May 2024 (The four-step 'playbook' the NHS uses to break whistleblowers) states in her survey that 16 out of 52 respondents were inappropriately referred to psychology/psychiatric services. However, it does not comment on occupational health referrals. There is statutory sick pay when one is unable to work, but the problem usually arises when asking for reduced hours or negotiating a "phased return". The advice from occupational health not to work excessive hours and have a guaranteed break at specified intervals looks promising on paper. But in practice, this often doesn't happen because of the staffing shortages. Some see the return of someone who has simply by their absence increased everyone else's workload (even if a locum is employed) as a bonus and 'use' them to fill the gaps, often unintentionally. This is a legacy of most of us who are conditioned to 'going the extra mile' every day, to complete our duties. The same conditioning makes the returnees feel guilty as well. Unless they are determined to stop work on time and or take breaks on time, no one is going to remind them unless they keel over in front of them or their patients!

It is not surprising then that around 45% of consultants are currently thinking of retiring in the next five years. The consultant workforce is not just ageing. Consultants are choosing to retire earlier than planned for a variety of reasons linked to job satisfaction, wellbeing, workload, ill health, bureaucracy and pension taxation rules[17]. A similar percentage of doctors in training are looking to work only part-time in the NHS or leave for work outside the NHS here or abroad, even leaving the profession for good. The BMA reported on a survey but on the ground, the juniors said it underestimated true intentions. Nine of out ten in one set said they would leave the NHS to go abroad or change careers.

A career in medicine consists of snakes and ladders. Snakes come in many guises as shown by the characters in the Charters and Mr Mayhem is often at one or more of the rungs of the ladder and invariably starts at the top one.

In the next chapter, I reveal how the rungs of the ladders can also become sabotaged.

Chapter 7

Snakes and Ladders 1995

My first substantive post was in Whitehaven Cumbria where the hospital had no cardiology service and patients had to travel over 120 miles across the Pennines to get diagnostic tests and treatments.

There was a small physician body of four and I was the fifth. Elderly care was better off with six consultants but declined to share the on-call medical take burden, preferring to run their own service and separate rota. I took over running the coronary care unit and upgraded the service provision in cardiology. I had already made plans to start local diagnostics quickly as the charity Heart Angina Support Group had funded a 'parking slab' and electricity access for the mobile catheter lab with technical staff and paid for ten visits. I recruited an experienced cardiac physiologist who I had previously worked with in Saudi Arabia and was at the time employed in the development and sales in Vingmed providing cardiac imaging echo machines and software. His wife also was a cardiac physiologist so gaining two in one go set up the department. We had a comprehensive echo service including transoesophageal echo (TOE), stress echo and an arrhythmia service.

Prior to my appointment in 1995, patients waited two years to see a cardiologist and now were seen in two weeks and whereas they waited years for a coronary angiogram (x-ray of heart arteries) there was now a fortnightly service of 12 cases. The impact was dramatic. I cleared the waiting list within the first 12 months. In addition to clinics at the local hospital, there was a satellite clinic in Workington.

James Ashman was my senior cardiac physiologist and kindly allows me to reproduce his reflections he wrote in 2003, following my sacking from Weston General Hospital.

Written extracts in 2003 by the Principal Cardiac Physiologist, at Birmingham Children's Hospital Cardiac Investigations Department.

I am a qualified Cardiac Physiologist with 21 years of experience in Diagnostic Cardiology working in NHS hospitals and Cardiac Ultrasound Industry (National and International Cardiac Specialist). I am currently the Principal Cardiac Physiologist. My training was undertaken in various places. When I completed my senior training, I moved abroad to Jeddah for financial reasons. It was here that I first met Dr Forbat. Dr Forbat was providing an echo service, and he required additional training in Doppler which I was able to provide him with. I was in Jeddah for three months and did not get to know Dr Forbat particularly well. However, after I left Jeddah Dr Forbat maintained contact. Dr Forbat was very well appreciated by patients. He was extremely committed and was very forthright and enthusiastic. He was meticulous and it is my view that others may at times feel threatened by him with his attention to detail.

Whilst I was working Internationally but living in Leicester, Dr Forbat approached me to see if I was prepared to set up a new cardiology department in Cumbria at the West Cumberland Hospital ("West Cumberland"). It was one of my career goals to develop a department. It meant a drop in salary but I was determined to take up the post. Dr Forbat and I shared a common ideal on how we wanted to involve people in the department.

West Cumberland had a fantastic charitable support base from which we were able to draw from and also Nyrex also supported the department. Looking back, I realise that the department was slightly spoilt as all things that were developed from scratch worked very well. There were occasions when Dr Forbat and I disagreed, but we were able to negotiate together to arrive at an appropriate decision. This was one of the things I admired about Dr Forbat. On arriving at Whitehaven, there were a few people already in the cardiology department. There was a combination of assistant technical officers, a part-time GP who carried out exercise tests but who had limited experience in interpreting the data.

When Dr Forbat left West Cumberland, the department had an additional echocardiogram lab with two echo machines and we were able to provide a regional echo service. Additionally, we managed to develop a paediatric echo service which we were able to use as a screening service. We also developed a pacemaker implantation service. The previous mobile cardiac catheter lab through charitable assistance led to the Trust paying for a fixed unit. We were able to persuade the Trust to appoint a second consultant in cardiology, Dr Wilmer. She provided a complimentary service looking at the rehabilitation side.

Dr Forbat also developed a transoesophageal echocardiography which allows the technician to identify foreign bodies in the heart that do not get picked up by normal ECGs. Additionally, there was a telemedicine service where we were able to transfer Echocardiographic studies to regional centres to avoid any unnecessary transfers.

I joined Dr Forbat in West Cumberland in 1995 a few months after he was appointed in post. On arrival, there was a huge backlog of people who had not yet been seen (about 500 patients waiting for echos). The closest geographical place for patients to receive an ECG was Newcastle. This meant that the disease of the local patients was much more severe than I would normally see. Dr Forbat was a pioneer for the GP open access service. This led onto a mobile GP open access echo service to cover the challenges of West Cumbria's Geography. I recall Dr X, a colleague of Dr Forbat, based at Carlisle was not supportive of this. Dr Forbat recognised, in my view, that patients needed this service and was prepared to develop a service to meet that need. Unfortunately, Dr X was openly hostile to the advanced development of services at Whitehaven feeling Carlisle with the larger patient centred population and didn't want the resources to follow the activity.

I am of the view that some people feel quite threatened about quality control and Dr Forbat was very good about that. I attended lots of meetings and Dr Forbat dealt with his colleague in one of those meetings when he was being aggressive and difficult to communicate with. Although Dr X was very opinionated and hostile, Dr Forbat treated him with a great deal of respect and in the appropriate manner.

I recall that at one time, we had a very short waiting list for cardio angiograms. Dr Forbat and I decided that an offer should be sent out to patients waiting more than 12 months in the Carlisle region to come to us for the procedure. Approximately 60/70 patients were approached and, of that, only 1 or 2 of that group agreed to come. I found that quite staggering. This fact was leaked into the local press when I was asked what Dr Forbat and I had achieved in Cumbria. There was a bit of an uproar about this and eventually more patients did come along for the service. It turned out that one of the first patients (who would have had a 12 month wait for an Angio if he had not come to West Cumberland) had a main stem lesion a critical lesion and if thrombosed was not survivable. I remember receiving a veiled threat from management about the disclosure I had made to the media.

I left West Cumberland two years after Dr Forbat moved to Weston Supermare. Just prior to me leaving West Cumberland, I trained up an assistant technical officer to a qualified physiologist. The Department, when I left, had 6 competent echo cardiographers which is more than most have in regional centres. In addition, there was an administrative assistant, a senior ATO, two trainees, and a part-time ATO. The Department no longer had a GP assistant because this was done through two staff grades and two consultant positions. The Department also had a colleague as a senior technician who basically undertook vascular services and therefore supported surgeons.

One of the things we tried to do was to give a service to all other departments. We both recognised that we deal with communities and it helps them to develop goodwill and that this could be done quickly in Cumbria so we allocated specific time for GP referrals or internal referrals. This avoided the situation where, if there was a long list, newcomers who needed to be seen quickly didn't have to wait.

All my trainees' reports were countersigned by a qualified technician. I do recall that starting a department meant that there was a battle to try and get the correct infrastructure in place, and I am of the view that that requires a lot of support and faith in the consultant and technical lead. Dr Forbat has always accepted criticism where I have drawn his attention to a misunderstanding, risk or human error.

I have faith in his clinical skill and judgment to recognise when things were not correct. This means that when you have a physician with no background in cardiology, they will make mistakes. Dr Forbat was not one of those consultant colleagues who was a law unto themselves. Dr Forbat should be able to talk freely and maturely to his peer colleagues. I always noticed good interaction and training, on the whole, was very appropriate.

Two years after I was appointed at West Cumberland the British Cardiac Society undertook a peer review as part of an agreed reciprocal arrangement with a similar DGH service.

British cardiac society peer review 9 September 1997
Following the visit on the 11th of November 96, by Dr E L Rose cardiologist at Halton General Hospital.

Strengths and innovative practices
Dr Forbat's abundant energy and enthusiasm for the post technical developments achieved in a short time pre-clinic nursing assessment one stop clinics good local chart will support there appears to be strong support for the cardiology services locally from local GP's and purchasers

Broad conclusions on the overall provision of cardiac services and training
I was generally very impressed with the achievements of doctor Forbat as a new consultant cardiologist having been imposed for only 18 months he has clearly been working extremely hard to develop cardiology services.

He has had a very clear dated goals which were based on careful assessment of local needs stop. His goals are about what he needs to develop and most of his success has been an improving service provision such as echocardiography, cardiac catheterisation and a specialist clinic. He has however fallen behind his goals a little in some areas which involve duplication of his influence so that he appears to be trying to do everything himself (i.e further progress is needed in terms of developing his team of junior doctors and technicians; Progress is also needed in terms of protocols and referral arrangements to reduce the amount of basic cardiological assessment that doctor Forbat is having to provide himself and thereby increases availability for more specialist assessment) Plans for collaboration with Carlisle should be encouraged.

Dr E L Rose

It became clear to my colleagues and the reason I was appointed was that I stood out as different, forward-thinking and energetic. I was fortunate enough to be supported by local GPs who at this time of fund holding were able to purchase services locally. *(See The Brotherhood – Patching in ceremony, see page 193.)* I was the first interventional cardiologist in Cumbria serving a population of one-third of a million, from Millom in the south to Carlisle in the north of the county. I rapidly built up a private practice due to demand and patients came from Carlisle to Whitehaven and even across the Pennines to see me. This was outside of my commitment to the NHS and I was working up to 90 hours including on-call one-in-five days and weekends. I started early and was never home early for our children and as soon as I arrived there would be phone calls for advice from colleagues on call. I would read to my youngest daughter before she went to sleep, but my wife often looked in to find I had dropped off with the unfinished storybook open on my lap! (See Episode 4, "Patch Over", see page 193).

Unbeknown to me when I arrived, one of the four physicians was under investigation regarding his clinical competence, in particular, in the management of cardiology patients when on call and covering the coronary care unit. This doctor had a good local network of supporters, notably extending to the regional centre where he trained, effectively one 'charter' within the Trust, so was somewhat protected from criticisms. This led to friction and breakdown in trust. I was soon to become aware of this, and it gave insight into the divide between adult physicians and those in elderly care. I realised that this played a part when it came to recognition of my work, as a single-handed cardiologist setting up a stand-alone local cardiology service from scratch, with close links to the regional centres across the Pennines. There was undoubted jealousy over my successful private practice, despite bringing in thousands of pounds a month to the Trust.

The local newspapers regularly had articles with me on the front pages, the first pacemaker implanted in Cumbria, the first coronary angiograms, etc. I naively expected recognition with some '*discretionary*' points. However, in my seven years I received not one. It is important to be aware of the process here. The committee controlled the process of allocation, so recommended these awards to the 'Charter', here comprised of surgeons and elderly care physicians who repeatedly award points to their own kind. They also voted to propose some of their colleagues for national C and B awards.

In joining the team, I was unaware concerns had been raised about a colleague's competence in my speciality of cardiology. The differences became even starker and consequently I was (wrongly) assumed complicit in raising concerns. Yet I was not made aware of this for the first year I was in post in an attempt by my colleagues to protect me from being involved. This was however an abject failure, as my peers informed me, notwithstanding the fact I had presided over one of the last cardiology units to be developed in a small district hospital in the UK.

Today, 20 March 2025, I received this testimony from Tahir Qaseem who moved on from Whitehaven to the United States.

Dr. Lance Forbat

It has been a true privilege to know and work alongside Dr. Lance Forbat over the course of my career as an internal medicine physician, gastroenterologist, and advanced endoscopist.

I first met Dr. Forbat when I joined him as a colleague at West Cumbria Healthcare NHS Trust between 1996 and 1999. At that time, I had recently completed my training in gastroenterology and internal medicine through the Harvard Medical School/University of Massachusetts system. My role at West Cumbria was to establish gastroenterology services and an endoscopy lab, addressing a critical shortage of acute medical services in the region. Similarly, Dr. Forbat was entrusted with the monumental task of developing cardiology services, including advanced procedural and interventional cardiology, at West Cumberland Hospital.

From the very beginning, I was profoundly impressed by Dr. Forbat's clinical expertise, his sharp diagnostic acumen, and his unparalleled dedication to patient care. He approached his role with a combination of technical excellence and deep compassion, ensuring that patients in this underserved community had access to the highest standard of cardiology care—something they had previously lacked. His ability to treat complex cardiac conditions with skill and precision transformed the healthcare landscape of West Cumbria.

What stood out most about Dr. Forbat was not only his extraordinary clinical skills but also his unwavering commitment to patient advocacy. He was driven by a vision to establish high-quality cardiology services for the local population, many of whom had previously been forced to travel great distances for specialized care. Dr. Forbat worked tirelessly to bring this vision to life, overcoming significant challenges such as funding limitations, resource shortages, and even resistance from administrative and institutional structures. Despite these hurdles, he remained resolute, rallying support from colleagues and demonstrating extraordinary perseverance in the face of adversity.

Throughout his tenure at West Cumbria, Dr. Forbat had multiple opportunities to leave for more lucrative or prestigious roles, but his devotion to his patients and his mission kept him rooted in the community. His impact was far-reaching—patients who once had to endure long journeys for cardiac treatment could now receive exceptional care close to home, thanks to the robust cardiology services he established.

I personally witnessed the profound difference Dr. Forbat made in the lives of our shared patients. His leadership, expertise, and compassion not only improved patient outcomes but also elevated the overall standard of care at West Cumberland Hospital. He is a rare and invaluable physician whose contributions continue to resonate long after his tenure.

It is with the highest regard and deepest respect that I offer my strongest support for Dr. Lance Forbat. His legacy as a physician, leader, and advocate for underserved communities is truly inspiring.

Sincerely,

Tahir Qaseem MD FACP FACG

In researching this further, I learned from my colleague consultant physician, Carl Thomson, the truth behind my suspicions. He wrote to me on 28th February, 2025;

"Dear Lance,

I have sifted through the papers on this, now almost 29 years old. ......

Oddly enough, it was only now after reading everything so many times that I think I have worked out the reasoning behind the Trust's decision to decline any significant action against our colleague. In one of his letters, the Chief Executive says that they have consulted the MDU and independent advisors who passed the issues as being within an acceptable level of clinical practice. Both John and myself were signed up with the MPS for professional indemnity while our colleague was in the MDU. He had been encouraged, I believe, by his advisors to canvass support from as wide a sample as possible, and this he did. I now think that it is possible that the trust and the MDU, including the other colleague involved, who later denied his initial advice to us, conspired to keep him in post to avoid enquiry into the cases by the public of his dismissal on grounds of incompetence became public knowledge. Both the trust and the MDU could then have faced some very expensive negligence claims. They already knew of my medico-legal work and perhaps my reputation among the lawyers for being honest and accurate.*

In retrospect, we should have, even at a later date, referred our colleague and the other colleague, to the GMC, but I guess that at the time John and I were at a very low ebb emotionally and professionally as a result of the loss of support from our colleagues which the management had aggressively fomented.

I look forward to reading more of your book, and happy to assist in any way.

Best wishes,

Carl"

* *John McCrea Rheumatologist and general physician (deceased) his family has permitted the use of his writing*

Despite our status as consultant physicians, were subjected to bullying. We challenged this and despite lack of response to representations by the HCSA to the Trust about bullying , we eventually raised our concerns at a meeting with the president of the Royal College of Physicians. Neither Carl, John, nor I received any awards. In my case this was despite a strong recommendation from the regional centre cardiologist who was Administrative Head of the Cardiac Catheter Laboratory, the National Audit Officer for the British Cardiovascular Interventional Society and Assistant Secretary to the British Cardiac Society!

Mr Mayhem was working hard in the background to prevent me from getting my recognition by the committee awarding points, despite support from my cardiology colleague in South Tees.

Reference for:
Dr Lance Forbat

From:
Dr MA de Belder MA MD FRCP Consultant Cardiologist
The James Cook University Hospital Marton Road
Middlesbrough TS4 3BW

I am a Consultant Cardiologist at the James Cook University Hospital, working in the Cardiothoracic Division. This provides tertiary cardiac services to a population of approximately 1.5million people, stretching from the west coast (Whitehaven) to the east coast (Hartlepool), as far north as Sunderland and Gateshead (and occasionally Carlisle) and down to Thirsk. I am Administrative Head of the Cardiac Catheter Laboratory and have direct responsibility for the interventional cardiology service. I have been the National Audit Officer for the British Cardiovascular Interventional Society for the last 5 years, serving on its Council for 8 years, and I am currently Assistant Secretary to the British Cardiac Society. I have a B merit award.

Dr Forbat was appointed to the West Cumberland Hospital in Whitehaven as a Consultant Physician with an interest in cardiology. For anybody going to this post, the easy route would have been to set up local outpatient services, advise on the guidelines to the coronary care unit and to develop a local non-invasive cardiology investigations service. Prior to Dr Forbat's arrival, cardiology services were provided either by a visiting cardiologist from the Freeman Hospital or by a locum.

Dr Forbat clearly set up all of these services but did a lot more besides. Knowing that the population of Whitehaven was disadvantaged geographically as regards access to tertiary services, he developed a number of services locally.

He developed one-stop out-patient clinics and built up the transthoracic echocardiographic services as well as providing a transoesophageal echocardiography service. He developed a trans-Pennine echocardiographic image transfer link so that he could discuss specific clinical problems with the regional centre cardiologists.

He initiated the cardiac catheterisation services by bringing in a mobile catheter laboratory as well as negotiating for a permanent cardiac catheterisation laboratory. He trained a number of registrars and staff grade cardiologists to help him run these services.

He developed a local pacemaker implantation service as well as a pacemaker follow-up clinic.

He recognised the importance of keeping up to date with interventional cardiology techniques and surgical techniques and travelled over to the James Cook University Hospital on a regular basis to have regular discussions with his regional colleagues. Clinically, he made a very sensible choice to investigate his unstable or sicker patients at the tertiary centre. He discussed patients who he felt should undergo revascularisation and shared the angiograms so that the most appropriate method was selected.

The effort that was required to develop all of these facilities was immense. He went about this task with formidable energy.

In addition, he had additional pressures by what appeared to be a chronic shortage of consultant staff at the West Cumberland Hospital. I suspect that he had to make a larger contribution to the running of the day-to day medical services than is delivered by many consultant physicians in this country.

It would be inconceivable to me that the huge effort that was required to develop these facilities for the benefits of the local population were not recognised by the process of distinction points.

Mr Mayhem also affected the three other physicians, but not the one under investigation who was awarded a C award. Eventually after working singlehanded for five years, 90 hours with pay on a 40-hour NHS contract, we appointed a second cardiologist.

A locum consultant wrote his assessment of the service that I inherited.

Dear Lance,

I thought I ought to drop you a personal note about my feelings regarding the current situation in Cardiology and General Medicine here at West Cumberland Hospital and offer you my wholehearted support for what you are trying to achieve. You have intimated to me on only a few occasions the political unrest that exists and the pressures under which you are working to try and provide the best possible Cardiovascular Service to this community. From what I gather historically you have made a significant impact over the last 4 years. I realise from my discussions with you that there are exciting plans for the future. In the very recent past I have become aware of some misgivings voiced by certain parties regarding Cardiology services. Obviously I am concerned since, having joined you, albeit temporarily. I am a provider of such services and the criticisms also reflect on upon my service. l have to say that I think the criticisms are totally baseless and have arisen from a complete lack of understanding and appreciation for the service that we provide. With the current resources I feel that we are doing everything possible to provide an excellent quality of service in as timely a fashion as possible. Increased throughput can only be further achieved by increased funding for equipment, technical, nursing and medical staff. To simply employ a second Cardiologist without the necessary support structure and to expect miraculous results is "pie in the sky" and reiterates a deep lack of understanding in all those who choose to criticise. One final point that I would like to make, which is related, is that I find it quite disturbing that management at the hospital don't appear to be supportive of your efforts. This is very divisive indeed. Progress cannot be made if there is no support. I hope this state of affairs changes for the better.

I support you without reservation and wish you luck in your endeavours.

Dr X.

I have now been in the second Cardiology Consultant position for almost 2 months, albeit without an actual second Cardiology firm. There has been criticism raised about the provision of Cardiology services and I would like to comment upon this, in particular the current practice of Cardiology and the potential to maximise such a service.

1) Outpatient Clinic (WCH)

The clinics at WCH are organised as "one stop" clinics which I believe is probably the most efficient way of seeing both new and old patients. The very nature of these clinics limits the numbers of patients that can be seen. Potentially more patients could be seen but this would require an increase in the number of senior physicians and technicians to process the increased numbers of patients. Space would be also important. Resources are very limited at present so increased throughput is impossible. The alternative is to increase the number of clinics at WCH - once again this would be impossible with the current state of affairs since the only times that clinics could be arranged would be Monday afternoons, Tuesdays or Fridays. The later 2 days are hooked up with invasive. non-invasive. and interventional procedures both at WCH and South Cleveland Hospitals.

Monday afternoon clinics would definitely interfere with general medical duties.

2) Outpatient Clinic (WI) – [Workington Infirmary]

Currently these clinics are not organised in the same manner as the WCH clinics, i.e. not "one stop" clinics. The number of new and follow-up patients is limited by the available time and this directly relates to the rather complex nature of cardiology patients and their problems

3) Technical Services

This includes echoes (adult, paediatric, open access), treadmill stress tests, Holters, stress echoes, and pacemaker services There is a large workload (inpatient and outpatient)with relatively minimal staff(ongoing staff training) and therefore long waiting lists. Ultimately this is a resource issue - not only with regard to provision of highly trained technical staff but also equipment and space to perform the procedures. Current resources are woefully inadequate I have been able to set up a weekly stress echo session. I have done this for 2 reasons - to perform viability studies and to try and not add to the lengthy standard treadmill stress test or the stress myoview waiting list. The maximum number of patients that can undergo this test in any session is 3 because of the length of the procedure With more technical staff, medical and cardiology nursing staff, space and equipment these sessions could potentially occur more frequently each week.

4) Cardiac Catheterisations

The number of cardiac catheterisation sessions has been increased to once a week and this has certainly reduced the waiting list. The number of patients on a list is limited by the available time An on-site facility with appropriately trained technical and nursing staff would provide a highly efficient service to optimise the delivery of such a service

5) Inpatient Cardiology

The standard of care for patients with cardiovascular problems varies enormously. This is to be expected when general physicians care for such patients. I don't feel that this is the optimal approach. Cardiologists seeing the majority of cardiovascular problems in the hospital would increase the inpatient workload exponentially but on the other hand there would be a much more uniform approach to patients and appropriate investigations and treatments could be implemented right from the outset as well as the use of the rather scarce resources (e.g CCU beds) Although unnecessary investigations would be prevented I think that the volume of procedures that would be generated would increase. A single Cardiologist in a busy district general would not be able to cope . with this change in practice and it may well be quite difficult for 2 whole time

Cardiologists to deal with the purely cardiovascular workload. It is a practice pattern that I believe in and would support. With regard to the CCU I feel that the number of beds are inadequate and their use by "all and sundry" sometimes quite inappropriate. I think there is a need for a pure CCU with haemodynamic monitoring and also a "high-dependency cardiac unit" with possible telemetry for the not so critically ill patient. This would allow cardiac patients to be looked after by cardiac nurses without the need to transfer to the ITU with its own limited resources. The nursing staff are excellent on the CCU and the acute medical wards but they would have to have additional training to allow for such a set up. Once again I don't feel that a single Cardiologist would be able to physically cope with this. Ultimately one has to have the best interest of the patient and this arrangement would, I believe, provide a high standard of inpatient cardiac care.

6) General Medicine Responsibilities
The general medicine workload is high with inadequate resources. Just concentrating upon the medical staff alone there is a lack of both senior and junior medical staff- the partial shift system has resulted in inadequate junior medical presence on the wards. Provision of an adequate medical service with cross covering issues is, and has been, quite time consuming. This obviously affects inpatient and outpatient cardiology service. A more efficient general medical service could not only be provided by increasing the number of junior medical staff but also having middle grade personnel e.g. specialist registrars.

7) Education
This is extremely important and always overlooked when service commitments are brought up for discussion. When I talk about education I not only refer to educating juniors but also continuing education for senior staff. It is very important, in my opinion, that one should be exposed to ongoing education and if this involves travelling to regional centres then this should be timetabled. This is the current situation. In my time here I have only been able to go to South Cleveland once! Part of continuing education involves keeping up ones technical skills be that angioplasty or electrophysiology. This can be achieved by

having strong links with a tertiary care facility at which one is able to perform these procedures.

In conclusion I feel that there is ample workload for 2 full time incumbent Consultant Cardiologists with the current set up. If all cardiology problems were seen by a Cardiologist and there was restructuring of the CCU as stated above then I daresay there would be enough work for 3 Cardiologists working full time providing an excellent uniform standard of cardiovascular care.

In order to provide an optimal service one not only requires the senior staff but there has to be an appropriate increase in support staff, equipment and space. Having senior staff alone would only result in increasing waiting lists for procedures and one is no further along. Criticism has been levelled against the Cardiology department in that waiting lists have not decreased significantly despite the appointment of a second Consultant Cardiologist. It is quite clear to me that the criticism stems from an inherent lack of understanding of cardiovascular practice in those people criticising the department and in those upholding these views. Not only is cardiovascular practice complex and time-consuming but simply increasing the number of senior staff without the necessary increase in support staff and equipment would not significantly decrease waiting lists. As it happens throughput has increased.

The general medical turmoil does not appear to be appreciated in terms of the additional workload both clinical and administrative.

In. my opinion the department is working at maximum capacity with the current resources available.

Dr X
Locum Consultant Cardiologist

I am also delighted to receive this feedback from a cardiothoracic surgeon working with my cardiology colleagues at South Tees NHS Trust.

Reflections on working with Dr Lance Forbat in the late 1990s

I started as a cardiothoracic surgeon at South Tees (South Cleveland) Hospital in 1994. This was a new cardiothoracic unit that was breaking the tradition of such units only being in major cities usually attached to established medical schools.

This new unit was part of the national strategy to meet the huge unmet need for cardiac care with the burden of disease mainly being suffered by lower income families in industrial areas, usually associated with tobacco smoking.

As cardiologists, surgeons, anaesthetists we were a (very) young group of enthusiasts who had learnt some of the new techniques being used to help these patients: percutaneous coronary stents; coronary bypass surgery; fast track recovery in intensive care. It was an exciting opportunity for us all as we had 'a clean slate' to introduce and adopt all the 'best' practices we had experienced in our relatively brief training.

It is worth remembering at this time that robust audit, quality assurance did not exist. Appointments were made on 'word of mouth' and brief interviews and higher specialty exams with evidence of training and attainment did not exist. Having said that we had a very good ethos of holding each other to account which meant we were well prepared for all the excellent measures that were subsequently introduced to assure high quality and safe patient care.

We were a very happy team excited to be delivering this relatively new care to the people of Teesside and beyond. And with our enthusiasm we were determined to use the cardiac catheter laboratory, cardiothoracic theatres and intensive care to the very limits of their potential – and we rapidly became national leaders (if not international) in this regard.

This is where Lance became such a strong addition to that service. On the west coast of the north of England there was a relatively 'neglected' population remote from centres of medical excellence. They had next to no cardiac care.

Lance arrived as a force for good and his achievements of the service he established in Whitehaven are well documented. Such achievements take huge energy, leadership and commitment. There is no doubt the population of Cumbria was most fortunate to have such a dedicated professional who had such a positive impact on cardiac care.

From my perspective it was a pleasure to work with Lance. I have to say I did admire him (as well as feeling sorry for him) as he only given access to the cardiac catheter lab at South Tees on Fridays. This meant that every week (after a full on four days in West Cumbria) he would drive over the A66 / Pennines in all weathers to arrive early to carry out the angiograms and stents for his patients. He would do a full day in the lab, which is intense work in lead aprons, and then make sure he found one of us as surgeons to discuss any potential patients who might need heart surgery. He would also handover any of his inpatients to the on call cardiologist at South Tees and then drive all the way back to West Cumbria in the evening – with all the traffic heading to the Lake District on what is well known as a dangerous road.

Lance was always positive and enthusiastic – such good attributes. And he clearly really cared for his patients and wanted them to do well. Great work and great achievements.

Simon Kendall
MD for Commissioning NW NHSE
Cardiothoracic Surgeon South Tees 1994 – 2022
President Society for Cardiothoracic Surgery 2020 to 2022

I was seven years in post before my wife could persuade me to move south nearer family and to be nearer my middle daughter, who was boarding at Millfield, having gained a swimming scholarship. This was a big decision as I had put my heart and soul into setting up the local service ***(see reference from John McCrea, sadly deceased 2014)*** including a vision to set up a sub-regional (satellite) cardiothoracic unit with encouragement from Graham Morritt, a senior surgical colleague in the tertiary centre in South Tees. I submitted a business plan helped by a cardiac surgical colleague in South Tees, which was blocked by the Chief Executive at the time (See Sound Words) No reason was given but this coincided with Tony Blair becoming Prime Minister and plans for the first PFI hospital to be built, not in Whitehaven where the service was most developed and pivotal to Cumbria but in Carlisle, which had very strong (political) links to the Freeman Newcastle Hospital. Whitehaven was not going to overcome this force (a key Charter) as fund holding was about to go, so removing the power from GPs and Whitehaven's continuing success under my leadership. Carlisle had also recruited a cardiologist a few years after my appointment, in doing so tipping the scales from the West to Carlisle.

Territorial lines had already been drawn up by the more powerful Charter with political backing at the highest level and sadly West Cumberland was going to suffer consequently. The die was set and I was looking to move. As a recognised leader it was hard to find a post that wanted my skills, as I was seen as a 'disrupter' in the minds of established units looking to appoint younger 'compliant' colleagues.

After dismissing an earlier advert for a hospital of similar size located on the western coast in the south, I was eventually persuaded to apply to Weston General Hospital, Weston-Super-Mare. I was more easily commutable to my wife's family in London and for mine in Surrey, and close enough to Millfield that my daughter could become a daygirl, and where subsequently my other two daughters would attend.

To attract me to the post and facilitate my move, I was offered waiting list clinics while I rebuilt a private practice to match what I left behind in Cumbria so I could cover my more expensive mortgage in the south and continue to afford the school fees. I was tasked to rebuild the local services using my experience and proven track record in Whitehaven.

References

John D McCrea MD (Hons) FRCP (Glas)

Ms Sonia Duckworth
Personnel Officer Medical Staffing
Human Resources Department
Weston Area Health NHS Trust
Weston General Hospital

Grange Road
Uphill
Weston-super-Mare
Somerset
BS23 4TQ
30 September, 2001.

Dear Ms Duckworth,

Re: Dr L N Forbat BSc (Hons) MD FRCP FRCP (Glasg)
I am honoured but also a little saddened to be invited to provide a reference for my colleague Dr Lance Forbat who was appointed as West Cumbria's first ever

Consultant Physician and Cardiologist in the spring of 1995 during my time as Clinical Director in General and Elderly Care Medicine.

During the last six years, Lance has built up a first-rate department both clinically and technically starting from scratch. He has provided a state-of-the-art echocardiography service including paediatric and transoesophageal echocardiography, full 24 hour ambulatory ECG assessment, a greatly expanded treadmill service (both with and without myoview imaging), "one stop" outpatient clinics, a permanent pacemaker implantation service, and a mobile coronary angiography service which will shortly be replaced by a fixed site angiography laboratory.

He has also secured additional funding from the NHS Regional Executive to provide a mobile echo service for North Cumbria. Last year his efforts to continue the momentum of cardiology development in the light of the requirements of the NSF and in cardiac rehabilitation lead to the creation of a second consultant post in cardiology.

Twice a month in all weathers Lance makes a round trip of over 200 miles to visit our local regional cardiology centre at South Cleveland Hospital Middlesbrough where he performs angiograms in patients with unstable angina. He also discusses patients from West Cumbria with the interventional cardiologists and cardiothoracic surgeons there

He has collaborated closely with his colleagues in South Cleveland Hospital to develop care protocols for a variety of cardiological conditions, thereby facilitating a seamless care network between the regional cardiology centre and the district general hospital. In addition, he has always shouldered a significant clinical load in general medicine and is on "emergency take" on a 1 in 6 rota.

The physicians, family practitioners and patients of this area owe him a debt of gratitude for his innovation, drive and vision. This has quite simply been to provide a first class comprehensive cardiology service to a part of the country with an exceptionally high prevalence of cardiac disease especially ischaemic heart disease. His clinical vision and continued commitment to service excellence in Cumbria lead the Royal College of Physicians and Surgeons of Glasgow to elevate Lance to the Fellowship qua Physician last month.

Despite the constraints in resources faced by everyone in the NHS in recent years, Lance is not easily discouraged and is not afraid of hard work. He has overcome many obstacles to develop a local cardiology service in Cumbria. His enthusiasm is infectious and his dynamism is always tempered by consideration for others coupled with a good sense of humour and an ability not to take himself too seriously.

Despite his technical prowess, Lance is also a very sound clinician and I place great reliance on his opinions which are always practical and sensible. I shall miss him both as a trusted and valued colleague and also as a friend.

He now wishes for completely understandable family reasons to move back to the south of England. I feel confident that he will enjoy working with new colleagues as part of a team and that he would enjoy the challenge of developing a superb cardiology service to meet your particular requirements. He has a proven track record in this field and can contribute a wealth of practical experience gained as a single-handed cardiologist in Cumbria.

I wish him and his family well but in the knowledge that our loss will be another hospital and surrounding community's gain. I can recommend him to you without reservation.

Yours sincerely,

J D McCrea MD (Hons) FRCP FRCP (Glasg)
Consultant Physician & Rheumatologist
Clinical Director General and Elderly Care Medicine (1993-95)

7th of May 2021

Carl Thomson
Qualifications: M.B. Ch.B. (Edin.) F.R.C.P. (Lond) F.R.C.P&S (Glasg.)
Retired NHS Consultant Physician GMC number 083315

I have known Lance Forbat since his interview for appointment as a consultant in West Cumberland Hospital in, I believe 1995, and worked closely with him in the medical department there until I left the hospital in 1999. Since then, we have kept in touch by correspondence and occasional meetings. Our last contact was in July 2020 when he took up a locum post in Carlisle and stayed at my home for one week until he found lodging near the hospital. During this time, over dinner conversations about medicine and his current work made it clear that he was knowledgeable and fully up to date with cardiology.

In the time that we worked together I was impressed by Dr. Forbat's clinical ability and decision making. Additionally he was always very quick to respond to a request to review a patient as part of his drive to good patient care. He was extremely energetic in setting up a full cardiology and angiographic department, as he had agreed to do when interviewed, and he did this by soliciting support from the community and charitable bodies. His pace in doing this sometimes pressurised the trust's management but the end result was a massive improvement to patient care as previously patients had to travel to Newcastle or Middlesbrough. He generated a prodigious workload but was loyally supported by his technical staff. In his work I would say that he was somewhat intense and driven, but only in the interests of meeting the clinical demands on the cardiology service. He is scrupulously honest and candid.

Carl Thomson

In January 2002, I moved to the Bristol area to take up my second single-handed post at Weston General in Weston-super-Mare. The similarities were there. The adult physicians were less numerous than the elderly care and there had been no substantive cardiologist for over six months.

Before my interview and to understand the challenge ahead (as I did prior to my appointment in West Cumberland Hospital) I arranged to meet several key people. The report on the Bristol baby scandal had just been published and Steven Bolsin, the anaesthetist who was the whistleblower had moved to work in Australia. With this knowledge, I met the Chief Executive Roger Moyse, Medical Director Dr Trisha Woodhead, Ian Baker, the head of Public Health Avon Health Authority. In my Palm V, I made notes of the meetings in preparation for the interview. (I continued daily entries during the year following my appointment and these were to be critical in evidence later on.) Clinical governance was high on the agenda following the Kennedy Report and a statement in parliament from Alan Milburn, then Secretary for Health (Bristol Royal Infirmary. Volume 378: debated on Thursday 17 January 2002).

The Kennedy Report, formally known as the "Report of the Public Inquiry into Children's Heart Surgery at the Bristol Royal Infirmary 1984-1995", was published in 2001[1]. It investigated the high mortality rates of paediatric cardiac surgeries at the Bristol Royal Infirmary and highlighted

The anaesthetist

DR STEPHEN BOLSIN was the first NHS whistle-blower to really hit the headlines when he highlighted the high death rates of babies having heart ops at Bristol Royal Infirmary.

His complaints led – after a long battle – to surgeons being struck off and a far-reaching inquiry.

Over six years he complained to hospital managers, then to the General Medical Council, and finally the Department of Health.

But far from being praised for highlighting dangerous practices, he was hounded out of the NHS.

The 49-year-old is now associate professor and head of anaesthetics at the Geelong Hospital near Melbourne, Australia. He moved there with wife Maggie, 46, and children Natasha, 16, and Christopher, 13 after being shunned by the NHS.

He says: "The effect on my family life and career has been profound and at times depressing.

Exile

"I am essentially a modern-day exile from the NHS. I could not get work within areas I wished to work in and could not stay in Bristol, where I was prevented from doing cardiac anaesthesia for some time and my work patterns were changed.

"The move to Geelong was a huge upheaval, which has fortunately worked out very well for us all.

"My children are now very Australian in their outlook and education but we all still miss aspects of UK life, particularly family."

Whistle-blowers such as Dr Bolsin are supposed to be protected from reprisals under Government legislation introduced three years ago.

All health authorities were ordered to appoint senior managers who staff could approach to raise concerns about malpractice without fear of being branded a troublemaker or damaging their career prospects.

The system clearly failed Dr Bolsin, who says the UK medical profession has still not formally acknowledged what happened to him.

But he adds: "Some senior doctors have told me confidentially that they admired my courage for speaking out. I'm not sure why they still can't speak out themselves.

"I believe that doctors must be able to go to trusted senior colleagues for advice if they believe wrongdoing is occurring.

"I have been, and still am, approached by doctors in the UK and Australia, and I admire the courage of many of these fine doctors who are still being forced to take the risks that I took six years ago to prevent patients from suffering unnecessary harm."

Dr Bolsin is adamant he would blow the whistle again. He says: "The answer is undoubtedly yes, if it prevented more children dying unnecessarily.

"My puzzlement has always been, 'Why didn't everyone else?'"

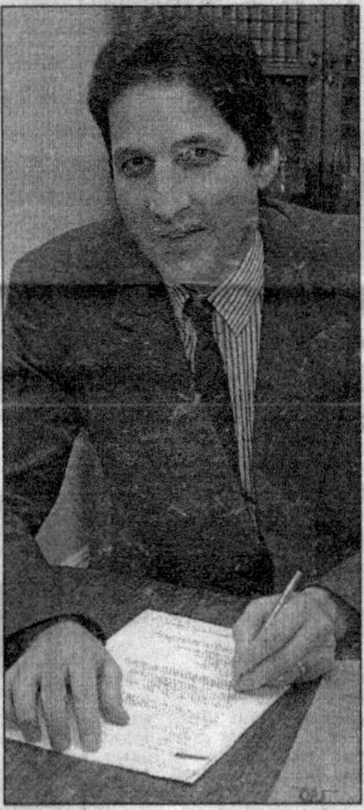

HOUNDED OUT . . . Dr Bolsin

The patient

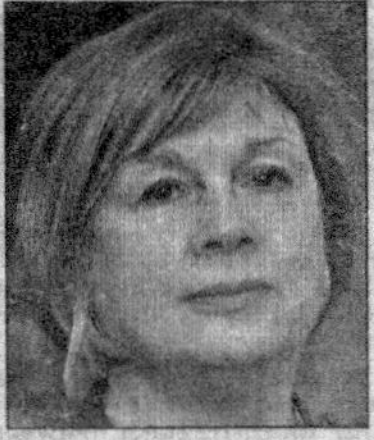

FORMER teacher GILLIAN BEAN'S heart disease was misdiagnosed for years then, when it was finally discovered, medics closed ranks and covered up.

Since she tried to complain about incompetent doctors Gillian, 60, has been refused treatment at her local hospital and is solely under the care of her GP.

This is despite her being on six heart drugs and having to retire due to ill health.

serious failings in the healthcare system that led to unnecessary patient deaths. Alan Milburn, who was the Secretary of State for Health at the time, responded to the findings of the Kennedy Report by acknowledging the failures identified and emphasising the need for reform in the NHS. Milburn's statement included a commitment to improving patient safety, transparency, and accountability within the healthcare system.

> *"The fault at Bristol, however, lay not with bad people, wrong though a few senior managers and senior clinicians were to act as they did. Underlying the whole Bristol tragedy was a much more profound structural and cultural problem—that of an NHS ultimately more geared to its own needs than to those of its patients, in which the question of accountability was confused in regard to services, professionals and patients."*

His government was prompted to take several actions following the report, including the development of new regulatory frameworks and the establishment of more robust mechanisms for monitoring the quality of care provided by hospitals.

I learned that a preliminary CHI report also highlighted deficiencies in infrastructure. There were poor information systems, limited multi-disciplinary audits, little progress in clinical risk management, recruitment and retention difficulties and lack of human resources staff.

I had concerns that there had been no cardiologist in post for over six months. I subsequently discovered clinical incidents that predated my start on 14 January 2002 and kept daily records (see appendix PIDA Flow sheet page).

There was no trained junior staff despite the nearby regional centre in Bristol. The previous consultant had retired early, *and I had my suspicion it may have been due to the increasing workload.* Much later, when I was raising concerns and experiencing difficulties making changes I wanted for a safe service, I contacted him to ask why he left. It became clear to me why on 21 October, 2022, after he replied by e-mail. The key points are summarised below;

> *'I gave one years notice. I had hoped to have a cardiologist before retiring.... This was partly due to tardiness on the part of the then medical director... The problem seems following the National Service Framework a large number of new posts were created and there were insufficient suitable staff to fill them... now choosing to apply for posts at a centre where they can carry out invasive procedures.... rather than such as at Weston where they are expected to do general medicine as well. The work just grew. I hope this is of some help to you.'*

I learned only after writing this chapter, that John passed away on 22nd April, 2019, aged 78, and left a message should his family want to contact me.

Chapter 8

Out on a Limb 2002

The Bristol Royal Infirmary Inquiry, also known as the Bristol Baby Inquiry, was a public inquiry conducted in the United Kingdom to investigate high mortality rates among infants undergoing heart surgery at the Bristol Royal Infirmary between 1984 and 1995 reported by Dr Stephen Bolsin cardiac anaesthetist. The final report of the Bristol Royal Infirmary Inquiry, chaired by Sir Ian Kennedy, was published on July 2, 2001, that vindicated his concerns and was a landmark in clinical governance. He subsequently found it impossible to find another position in the UK and moved to Australia.

Cardiology Department Weston General Hospital 2002:
When I arrived on my first working day expecting my induction, the timetable did not consider that a. I had an outpatient clinic, b. I was rostered as the consultant on call for acute medical take, and c. I had no junior or senior SHO. In my first six months, this was my assessment of the service I inherited:

1. *No full-time qualified technician and when there were two part-timers, there was no overlap between technicians and my timetable as their overlap was the day I am at Bristol. No one present at all on Fridays!*
2. *No data base in department.*
3. *No records of test results for ETTs, ECHOs or 24-hour BPs. Only 24-hour tapes on the Reynolds database.*
4. *No tracer system for results*
5. *Substandard tests procedures and protocols.*
    a. *No diaries requested with 24-hour tapes, wrong settings on Exercise Test protocols (under review).*
    b. *Untrained ATOs doing ETTs.*
    c. *Untrained MTO doing ECHOs unsupervised majority of time.*

6. *Absent staff grade for the last four of the six months I have been in post. It is clear from cases reviewed that this staff grade was not adequately trained in ETT or ECHO and was inappropriately left unsupervised.*
7. *No cardiologist overseeing department at all for six months prior to my arrival.*
8. *No audit of activity or quality control.*
9. *Old equipment requiring review and ECHO equipment for bought for £50,000.00 in absence of cardiologist in post, which is unsuitable for the development requirements of department. (Senior cardiac physiologist's comments to follow.)*

Out-patient service:

1. *No structure on arrival, height, weight, ECG, CXR etc.*
2. *No one-stop facility despite impressions given.*
3. *Poor x-ray service with slow turn around. X-rays unreported.*
4. *Follow-up clinic too full, 32 patients in morning.*
5. *Planning poor with ad hoc urgent new patients added on.*
6. *Due to lack of cardiologist, follow-ups from previous general physician locum review actually require time as a new patient.*
7. *Over 50% can be discharged as I apply my usual practice. The time required to educate and explain to patients used to yearly follow-up.*

I assessed the workload including the backlog due to there having been no cardiologist for over six months prior to my appointment. This is the summary I documented at the time:

> *"Based on my experience I calculated the backlog would require a minimum of 3 weeks to sort out. I requested 3 weeks out of medicine to set up the service, address training and clinical governance issues, but mainly to catch up with the backlog of reports and letters (over 140 in January at last count). From the outset I have been running a general medical firm with depleted junior staff, covered a 3 week absence of a colleague in elderly care, yet I have had insufficient and intermittent (and some incompetent) secretarial and technical support throughout. Whilst trying to revive the cardiology service I have had to manage without full time or fully trained technicians and the last 8 weeks an absent staff grade in*

cardiology. I have reduced inpatient waiting for angiography from 3 months to one week, but the rest of the service is building up behind me. I have also seen 6 month waiters in general medicine and cardiology when my private clinics were light at the start of my job."

It became evident to me shortly after I settled in that my assessment was conservative and outpatient clinics were overbooked and unmanageable, with long waiting times and there were several filing cabinets with unreported investigations up to a year old. I was part of the on call one-in-five medical rota and requested I come out of this to cope with the enormous cardiology backlog and time for development of the service. Soon after, I was informed of complaints about my service to the medical director. I wrote to the Medical Director Dr Trisha Woodhouse in support of my case:

"I am particularly concerned by your comment that I might be the subject of a complaint to the GMC because of incident forms submitted regarding me arriving late at a couple of clinics. This was perceived to be a consequence of my private clinic overrunning, when in fact my delay was overrun due to dealing with NHS problems during the scheduled private clinic★*. You also said that 'people' could say I am behind with referral letters and reporting despite the agreement that there is the workload for 2 cardiologists, with full supporting staff (not there) and not because I am in my private clinic (sessions were agreed before was appointed). The NCAA was the last option (confirmed in a letter from Sir George Alberti when PRCP).*

In addition many of the junior doctors employed by the Trust were not all British trained graduates and lacked experience and often ability. Very early on I raised my concerns about poor patient care.

We have a meeting 09.00-11.00 on 1st July with Sean Cusack from the BMA to discuss my job plan and I suggested Dr X join us as he is lead physician and there is no clinical director. I would like to ask again for your support in providing the time and resources I have requested to deliver the cardiology service."

★ Juniors were sent to interrupt my private clinic sessions with non-urgent problems that should be dealt at the ward rounds.

A locum agreed I could make a recording of his experience, as an independent observer, but was afraid to be identified for fear of reprisals: I have copies on two audio CDs confirming that there were major deficiencies in the quality of juniors and that many incidents occurred. *He also made it obvious that ward rounds were longer due to re-checking everything. In addition, he was not consulted as a senior member of the team and ignored by a Senior House Officer until I intervened.* An alternative view was given by the Trust where notes were made following a call from the same locum apparently saying ' ... *not pleased with lengthy ward rounds' ... and 'Dr Forbat is not a very confident physician' and 'the extra paperwork he asks for is a waste of time.'* This was disconcerting for me, as these comments did not reflect his clear concerns spontaneously raised with me. Indeed, in another statement from an SHO, who worked with me for six months in 2002, wrote '*I interacted with him well. If I had any problems, then I would ask Dr. Forbat... It is the nature of Dr Forbat to do things quickly. He did do filing...probably trying to set a good example. I found him more approachable than Dr X (*another consultant) *and I do not recall hearing anything about Dr. Forbat'.*

Nothing changed and I collected evidence and regularly submitted Datix forms (documenting near misses or actual harm to patients) in the belief that after the Bristol scandal, raising concerns as a doctor (a duty of candour) would be seen as a positive contribution to patient safety. In my PIDA Flowsheet (example in appendix) I kept detailed records of events in my Palm V and PIDA flow sheet, I have kept for my reference, including incidents of patient harm or preventing potential harm, governance issues, bullying and harassment, job plan issues and staffing shortages. I made contemporaneous entries from 1st October 2001, before my appointment and first day on 14th January 2002, up to when I was sacked on 30 December 2002 and continued to 22nd January 2003, whilst waiting for the draft report from the NCAA. On at least seven occasions I had inadequate or no technical service, eight echo cases of incorrect reports, inappropriate or misinterpreted exercise tests, 43 concerns on management of patients, 13 errors to administration of medical records. I requested review of my job plan on 29 occasions (as advised in the Royal College of Physicians guidelines18) with only once a positive response, on six occasions there were major gaps in junior or consultant cover where I was ultimately responsible, I recorded 39 episodes where I felt bullied and at least five complaints I had to challenge as they were falsely or wrongly assigned to me.

At the time I arrived on the scene (and sadly even then in 2023) my experience raising concerns was not welcomed. My error in retrospect was to raise several Datix reports in any day and discuss my concerns with my immediate manager (See Appendix the HCSA Playbook). I was also reducing clinics to manageable numbers and doing extra angiogram sessions to clear the backlog, which the purchasing GPs had funded to be performed on NHS patients at the private BUPA hospital. (See Episode 5, see "Giving Back", page 183).

I was now a problem to the Charter. I realised I was being sidelined in things I should have been involved in. I learned that one secretary (Tara Knowles) was married to a consultant, who, amongst others, was keeping tabs on my movements, as when in a lunchtime break, I was signing my NHS letters in the private wing, the only quiet office I could find without being disturbed! I had been in post three months and only later I learned that behind the scenes I was being undermined by *Tig Trager* (Consultant A), *Bobby Manson* (Clinical lead) and *Harry (Opie) Winston* (Nurse) and plans were underway at the *'Reaper Table'*, with *Clay Morrow* (CEO Roger Moyse) plus *Jax Teller* (Medical Director), *Bobby Manson* and *Chuck Marston* (Finance department) likely players to be present round the table, deciding on a strategy how to remove me from my post (some months after my sacking, CEO Roger Moyse was sacked for fiddling waiting lists for bonus payments, whereas *Clay Morrow* was replaced by Jack Teller) so I know my restructuring of clinics also played a role here. I was summoned to a meeting in the Bristol Royal Infirmary and raised my concerns with the cardiology lead, making what I believe was a protected disclosure. I voiced my opinion that I was working in a culture akin to that described in the recently published Kennedy report on the Bristol baby scandal. I was told by *Jacob Hale Jr* (professor of cardiology) in no uncertain terms to 'back off'. I don't know if he was warning me to protect me or was part of the Charter. Similarly, I can only surmise the motives *Jax Teller* (medical director), who was well behind this and had already told me not to look at past and present problems and get on with the backlog. My request for notes (all paper records) to enable me to review the unreported tests was also refused. I next went to see Mike Durkin at the Strategic Health Authority with my concerns. The outcome was not helpful. He did not set up a meeting between me and Trust as I had hoped.

I also wrote to the BMA:

"Regarding the proposed job plan starting next week, you will see from yesterday's e-mails,

a. there was a total lack of outpatient support with inadequate notes preparation and lack of results. The nurse running the clinic was very supportive and wrote on the time sheet that there were problems with each patient. It will not be possible to run to time even with the proposed reduction in number. Also no-one is yet allocated to reorganise the clinics before Thursday! I had no technician, away again next week.

b. the juniors inexperience and lack of numbers (one senior SHO down) means that 30 patients cannot be seen safely in a 3 hour ward round. One example was the patient in whom I replaced a chest drain at 19.30. At the start of my clinic I rang my SHO to the locum agency 'senior SHO' (who is even more junior) and asked to see the x-ray in clinic as I didn't want a problem again at 17.30. She said the x-ray had been done about an hour earlier. When I saw it the lung had deflated and the tube was perfectly placed. There was a lung leak requiring a low pressure pump. I asked her to get on and if necessary speak to a thoracic surgeon at the BRI. Also I suggested she get the x-rays reported and show them to a chest physician as I didn't want the patient left in limbo over the weekend. I heard no more and rang at 17.30. The locum SHO said the chest physician (name redacted here) had seen x-rays and confirmed drain perfectly placed by me and that a low pressure pump was needed. The SHO said no-one knew what pressure to set the pump and the thoracic surgeon was in theatre at the BRI and not replied. She was just going off duty and said she was about to ring the on call SHO to deal with the pump! This is my current SHO who I have never seen put in a drain and from my teaching clearly had not been taught properly. The locum had not spoken to the nurses on the thoracic ward at BRI. I asked her to ring ward 5a at BRI before she went home and find someone who could advise our surgical ward nurses. I rang 19.00 and problem resolved with help from nurses on the respiratory ward.

c. *secretarial efficiency: they need a lot of support. I could have done 90 minutes dictation after signing letters, instead of 2 hours checking and correcting letters.*

And followed up:

"I need advice on how to proceed with the new job plan if this continues.

My intentions: to develop a first class cardiology service in Weston as I did in Cumbria and forge strong links with the regional centre to develop my career. I want a colleague at Weston I can trust and await response to advert for the second cardiologist with closing date 12.07. My senior technician starts 22.07 and will be a major ally and asset.

I would like to make this career move to Weston work as the option of another move is not on. I required equity in my treatment in the Trust. The Trust has just appointed an Elderly care physician who was in private practice and had an academic background. The consultant had references suggesting concerns about her ability to do acute general medicine. They had been appointed but will not do any acute medicine for the first month until 'settled'. Then the consultant may join a supervised on call with a senior colleague shadowing her!! This is ridiculous. Here I am 6 months without any support or time to settle in and resolve the cardiology mess and back-log, very experienced (I would argue more than any of the other physicians at Weston!) and being bullied, sneered at, harmed and now under review by colleagues that cannot be trusted!"

I became suspicious of who might be orchestrating this. One thing troubled me as I recalled what Professor Gianni Angelini told me soon after my appointment. I spoke with him recently and as two decades had gone by since my appointment, I had to remind him of what he said to me. I refer to contemporaneous notes made on my Palm V device. He informed me of a call prior to my interview from someone trying to block my appointment, but he declined to tell me the source at the time. I wrote that Gianni said that it was an 'unsolicited' e-mail or phone call to Weston General and he had persuaded me to get some referees to phone in my support. The person said, "they were not from my hospital" and words to the effect, "not to employ Dr Forbat as he was a troublemaker and did little work." Gianni confirmed this, "*on recollection, it was from West Cumbria, possibly somebody from the hospital you were working at. There is no way I could remember the name. It could not have been from Bristol because the Bristol trainees were not interested in it and were reluctant to go to Weston because of the mess with the service.*" He also said from his perspective at the BRI, the cardiology service was significantly better after my arrival.

I find it incredible to think such a call/e-mail would be made and suspect it originated from West Cumbria (a Northern Charter).

I have since wondered if my Mr Mayhem was prepared to do anything to undermine me, for exercising good medical practice (GMP) and the 'duty of candour', i.e. "to speak out if any concerns related regarding bullying or substandard patient care every doctor is expected to uphold"?

On 10 January, 2003, I was listening to radio 4 around noon and there was discussion about the finance director at St George's Hospital and whistleblowing with Mrs Myers, deputy director of PCAW (Public Concern at Work) and it jogged my memory of a meeting Sean Cusack (BMA) and I had with Dr Woodhead, and John Edwards (HR) on 22.10.02.

I made a note in my Palm V, 2002-07-04 00:13

> *"Trisha complained that I had taken my concerns about serious clinical incidents outside the trust (i.e. whistleblown) to Mark Outhwaite at the SHA (meeting 29.08.02 and letter 03.09.02). Dr. Woodhead said Mike Durkin was following these up. Sean said that the trust had moved outside the trust first by referring me to the NCAA. I believe this reinforces the reasons why I have been sacked. All my e-mails before I arrived revolved around a workable timetable and clinical governance issues (see e-mails October -December 2001) and after arrival the lack of staff further compromised a workable job plan and quality of patient care. The latter was the theme throughout (and commented by Mrs Myers on Radio 4)."*

The following exchange of e-mails confirmed to my mind that I was being sidelined…:

> *"Following Roger Moyse's instruction to prevent the PCT sending me waiting list work at the Glen I enclose e-mails from M of the PCT. She is aware I am forwarding them to the HCSA and BMA."*

Lance,
Have sent an email which I hope will help. Be assured of my support through this trying time.
With best wishes
M

Dear Dr Forbat,
As requested, I am writing to inform you of the following instructions I have received from Julie Sharma, Chief Executive, North Somerset Primary Care Trust.
The situation to date is that the PCT has been formally asked to slow down the waiting list initiative on the basis that there appears to be issues unresolved with the Weston Area Heath Trust and yourself. Exactly what issues have not been divulged to me personally.
However, I have been in contact with Julie Sharma this evening and she has informed me that she will write to you formally regarding the situation.
I realise this outcome is disappointing for you and I feel the same as I have no doubt that both of us were putting patient care first.
Yours sincerely
M

In my sixth month I went on holiday and when returned on the weekend I had a letter from the Trust. The letter sent to my home while I was on leave had invited me to attend a meeting with the Trust management. No reason was given, however, the letter said not to enter the premises, and I suspected it was something serious. Without relaying the content to my wife, I decided anyway to go in on that weekend. My concerns were to see if anything had been disturbed in my office, to see the backlog of work I left behind before my holiday and if I could clear some before Monday. It was evident the Charter had been ready for my return, weekend or not. I assume I was seen entering the department and as I came out of my office a security guard accosted me and said I was not allowed in the building and escorted me out of the hospital. This was the start of my 'garden leave'.

The BMA was unable to help or any of my colleagues in the Trust prepared or willing to support me, no doubt under strict instructions from managers. This is a tactic I came across again two decades later in a locum when my chaperone in my outpatient clinic promised to give me a statement to counter a complaint by a patient but withdrew this offer when she told me she was threatened by management with potential disciplinary action if she wrote a statement in support of my account.

As I gathered more information about charges the Charter had raised against me it was abundantly clear to me that over the previous three months, a case was being built against me. I was referred to the then NCAA (National Clinical Assessment Association, subsequently renamed NCAS) for 'underperforming' doctors, having failed earlier to get a review by the BCS in support of my concerns about the workload and deficiencies in the service I inherited. The Trust had to invite BCS on behalf of the Trust and they declined and it was obvious to me they did not want outsiders independently reviewing the service.

Doctors Net News December 2003: Rules May End Suspension Scandal

New procedures will help put an end to the scandal of doctors being suspended for months and years at a time, it was claimed yesterday. Doctors should only be suspended for four weeks at a time, according to a new Department of Health framework.

The new rules say that a doctor's first exclusion from work should be for no more than two weeks and subsequent extensions no more than four weeks.

It calls for employers to use better case management and to conduct quick and thorough investigations, all under the supervision of a board member.

It says that when a doctor is not referred for disciplinary or capability procedures, a programme for return to work should be put in place.

The chief medical officer Professor Sir Liam Donaldson said: "This will see an end to the kind of situations that occurred in the past where patients were left unprotected because no-one was sure how to deal with a doctor with performance problems.

"It will also be good for doctors with emphasis on early intervention to provide support rather than disciplinary action late in the day. It should also see an end to the long suspensions culture of the past."

Mr Nizam Mamode, chairman of the BMA's consultants and specialists negotiating committee, said: "This agreement is a significant initial step along the way to addressing our concerns that suspensions are misused.

It is my belief the Trust was minded to conclude that I was incompetent, easily achievable by giving me an impossible workload (see reply to NCAA below), without support (no notes, no protected time etc) and trawling for anything in support of the case they were building. But to my mind the fact that I had raised concerns (which I consider protected disclosures) was in the eyes of the Charter a threat to their reputation, especially after the Bristol baby scandal publication.

I refer again to the supporting letter from Colin Dyan working both the BRI and Weston General Hospital:

> *"I remain convinced, as I mentioned in a previous e-mail, that the best way to resolve the situation and achieve some success in the cardiology service would be to relieve Lance of his General Medical duties for a significant period of time (e.g. 3 months). If following this he has not managed to make inroads into the cardiology backlog then it would seem appropriate to be concerned about his management of the service. Until then it will tend to be one opinion against another. I am aware that I am in a minority of the physicians in this view and can only speak personally."*

and this reply to NCAA from the appointed cardiologist assessing the report:

"Dear xxxxxx
My comments on the Trust's response:

1. There is a major professional difference between the previous post holder who did no invasive work and Dr Forbat's post which involved being offsite a whole day per week doing invasive Cardiology.

Dr Forbat had 3 components to his job – acute general medicine takes and follow up of these patients - single handed running a DGH cardiology department - cardiac catheterisation at Bristol Royal Infirmary

I think Dr xxxxxxx agrees that this is an ill-judged job plan and I am sorry that the Trust seems unwilling to acknowledge this.

2. I may have missed it in the paperwork, but I don't believe that the Trust previously, or now, have made the simple transparent statement that the Cardiac Department should have two Consultant posts and has never been" single handed."

<u>From: Head of Technical Services Cardiology Department 18 December, 2002</u>

To whom it may concern

Being aware of the current investigation by the NCAA of Dr L Forbat Consultant Cardiologist it seemed to me to be appropriate to offer some sort of impartial view of my time since arriving at the Weston General Hospital Cardiology Dept.

I was appointed Technical Head of Cardiology arriving in July of this year as a measure to improve the technical services. My reasons for coming were partly family-orientated but largely due to the forward thinking ideas and competence of Dr Forbat, of whom I had come to know through my brief stay at the West Cumberland Hospital, where he was very popular with my fellow technical colleagues. Having spoken in great length with Dr Forbat before my arrival at Weston I was fully aware of the necessity to promote and enhance the cardiology service. His vision and enthusiasm paralleled my own views and with this in mind made my decision to move more exciting. Interestingly the Weston management appeared to share the same vision.

It was with a great sense of disappointment, that his early, " suspension from duty" following my arrival made life extremely difficult. Having now been in post for 6 months I feel fully justified in offering an opinion about the problems, I believe he endured.

Obviously I am not immune to many of the rumours and accusations surrounding his position, many of which I believe to be totally unfounded and largely borne out by ignorance of the intense workload and pressure he was subjected too, for which my department was largely at fault.

From a technical base I can only describe practices and technical competence in the department as basic, and lacking in experience. In the very short time I spent working with Dr Forbat at Weston, I was asked by him to review a number of patients technical results, which he seemed to find confusing. In all instances, I had to repeat these tests to support his clinical findings. What was patently obvious to me was that technical information was sub-standard, and had been over many months/years that records showed. One could argue that lack of continuity of staff i.e locum cover, or inadequate training was at fault, but the result was a constant double checking of earlier history with regards to patient tests, which resulted in a slowing of patient throughput.

I have attempted to redress this issue since my arrival and have received a lot of support from management and staff at Weston. We are however still without a cardiologist on site. It bemuses me totally that such a competent cardiologist as Dr Forbat, who's skills in this area I greatly admire and who's temperament under intense pressure was admirable has found himself in the position he is in.

I can only assume, the breakdown in communication between Dr Forbat and management was by circumstance. As both parties appeared shared the same vision.

Yours Faithfully

Head of Technical services Cardiology Department

'The above letter I'm happy to stand or fall by as I believe it to be true, and if necessary accept if management get to read it. Comments about your secretary and individual staff and how you are perceived, again I would comment on if interviewed.

The above letter I believe I can defend and they shouldn't take offence at, and if they do well sod it.'

I contacted David in December 2023, 21 years later asked him if still vivid in his memory to recall his time at Weston General prior to my arrival, my impact on the service and his observations of other staff during my brief tenure and the aftermath following my sacking;

"Speaking from a technical viewpoint it was very clear that tests and procedures fell well below expectations, this was probably understandable given all of the technical cardiology staff were not qualified to undertake many of the tasks for which they were assigned.

This led too many mistakes and misinterpretation of results.

At this time prior to my arrival they were supported by consultant with an interest in cardiology and a staff grade GP, working part time.

Following this persons retirement a newly appointed cardiologist (LF) was employed to not only take over the service, but also to reduce a substantial backlog of patients.

Serious misgivings about some cardiology diagnoses during this time were brought to my attention, by LF on my arrival, and having read some of them it was obvious things were not quite right.

There was a substantial delay between the retirement of the previous consultant and the new appointee, to which it can only be assumed that mistakes would have been more likely prevalent during this time period.

I don't believe it is within my scope to apportion blame, but it was my belief that the medical support for cardiology patients at this time was poor.

To this end and give the constraints of time the new consultant would have had little choice, but to bring this to management's attention, exactly how this was done, I am not in a position to comment but issues he would have raised would have made for very uncomfortable reading for those involved in some of the diagnoses, during this interim time period."

... "given the strong personalities involved, there was a major kickback from a collective group of consultants, who were involved in the interim cardiology decision making, added to this was the assistant technical staff who were also left wanting.

For me the problem LF faced was ruffling feathers and embarrassing too many people, both medical and technical.

LF from my perspective was a very hard working conscientious experienced cardiologist, who also devoted many hours outside of the routine to try and make up for the backlog.

It did not take long for management to hit back, and as I saw it, there was a concerted effort to drum up as much support as possible to label him as erratic and unsuitable for the position. As is usual in the case of those in control, there will always be a long list of supporters to support the management line, for their own personal gain.

As far as I was concerned all were complicit in poor practice, this was something I pointed out at the GMC (corrected NCAA) body interview, I was asked to attend. It would seem I was a lone voice.

What followed was his suspension and subsequent removal. This was not only an incredibly difficult time for LF, but to a lesser extent myself.

Following the arrival of a hastily appointed Locum cardiologist, we were still left with a horrendously large backlog of patients, which were known to contain a number of misdiagnoses.

Management at this time decided to send all the backlog of patients back to the relevant GP's for re assessment and re-referral, allowing the new locum a clean slate of patients. It would be approximately another year before a fulltime cardiologist was employed and soon after a second cardiologist.

Interestingly from what I remember, he (JE) proposed to do exactly the same things as the first cardiologist (LF) only in this case he had a tremendous amount of support, notably from the soon to arrive second cardiologist. I myself also followed up with 2 more experienced physiologists and a trainee."

......."you got stitched up by the collective group of consultants, who wanted you out for embarrassing them, a load of assistants technical staff who were not trained, but thought they were, and a load of nurses on the wards who didn't like your out of hrs ward rounds."

It is interesting here to note the similarity to the initial reaction to the development of West Cumberland Hospital cardiology services and the expectations of the Trust highlighted in the review by the locum cardiologist; '*lack of understanding and appreciation for the service that we provide. With the current resources I feel that we are doing everything possible to provide an excellent quality of service in as timely a fashion as possible. Increased throughput can only be further achieved by increased funding for equipment, technical, nursing and medical staff. To simply employ a second Cardiologist without the necessary support structure*'

Patients would be unaware of the poor clinical decisions and that these were covered up. Those coming to harm would never know the reason or that I was trying to prevent further mistakes and potential harm. Patients were not diagnosed correctly or even if diagnosed not referred for surgery in a timely manner. Those coming to harm will never know that I was sacked for raising these concerns!

I was being punished for exercising my duty of candour to protect my patients. I sought advice from the MPS, HCSA and Public Concern at Work (PCAW see their report May 2013) on the PIDA law[5], but it became clear PIDA had no teeth. I was alone at home, going into debt without my private income relying on the basic NHS salary. I got up each day, as if for work, so maintained a routine to occupy myself. My time was divided between building evidence to defend my position and converting my loft into another room. Knocking a wall through into my loft with a sledgehammer was a therapeutic action and an outlet for my anger and sheer frustration with my predicament.

When the assessment by the NCAA went ahead that November, I had all my evidence and backers from Cumbria to counter the local Charter's attack on my professionalism and clinical competence. I had to undergo a series of simulated clinical scenarios (akin to undergraduate OSCE's – objective structure clinical assessment) where actors played the roles of patients and staff, something new to my generation of consultants and I had no idea this would not be the first time I would experience this. A series of interviews followed and then a long wait for the outcome. It soon became clear to the Charter this was taking a long time, and the report was not expected until the following January or February. I went on holiday over the Christmas New Year break with the children to our timeshare in Spain. On my return and opening my mail, there was a letter from *Clay Morrow* (Roger Moyse) informing me I had been sacked. The reason was abundantly clear to all. If they waited beyond January 1st for my report, I would have full employment rights due attaining to one year of employment (in 2002, the previous seven years as a consultant in the NHS did not count as accrued with a with different Trust) and could have lodged a claim for unfair dismissal with a tribunal. Sacking me was the Charter's solution to this predicament and so to avoid any publicity. There were threats to refer me to the GMC and indeed it was after the NCAA report cleared me of incompetence. The only things they managed to make stick with the panel was to convince them I should attend a course on 'time management' (ignoring the impossible workload without any support!) and an 'anger management course'. The NCAA staff were very supportive:

"Dear Lance

Further to my email below - I have now checked whether the 20 courses are suitable and I am pleased to confirm that they are. I am also happy that you contact Mike Durkin direct to ask him to fund the courses. Could you copy this email to him so that he has confirmation from the NCAA to do this. You will have to discuss any compensation for lost income with Dr Durkin directly.

Alan Swain Senior Casework Manager"

However, I could not help but be disappointed by the NCAA as I felt it had not paid sufficient attention to my claims against the Trust and the evidence I had produced in support of my position. I was a whistleblower and the Charters knew how to circumvent this, as investigating the PIDA laws, I learned they were often ineffective. I felt I had nowhere to go, no life raft and the outcome (and was in retrospect predicted) under duress from both parties. Most reluctantly, I agreed to a settlement, which was of comparatively very little value, especially with the detrimental effect it was going to have on my future and that of my family. I was confronted with a 'gagging clause (*in retrospect expected* and *now illegal in the NHS)*.

The CQC inspected Weston General Hospital in June 2021 and rated the core service inadequate. In the 2005/2006 period on the quality of the healthcare it provided, the hospital was rated as weak on a four-point scale of weak, fair, good and excellent. This placed the hospital in the bottom performing 9% of trusts in the country. On the same scale, the hospital's use of resources was also rated weak, placing it in the bottom 37% of trusts in the country.

On 7 July, 2003, BBC Television programme Inside Out broadcast allegations from a whistleblower that senior management within the hospital were putting pressure on employees to manipulate waiting list statistics to make them look more favourable. An independent enquiry in 2004 concluded that this manipulation did take place.

Readers may find it difficult to understand the stress endured and how my family and I felt during this period. There was stress at work and at home. Every time I came home from work and told my story to my wife, I relived the problems with emotion and if a locum job ended earlier than expected, even if for a simple money-saving reason by the Trust, it was me who was deemed to be at fault. Consequently, arguments were common and I was frustrated and feeling unsupported. I could not win and often internalised events and did not discuss my day. All of you unnamed whistleblowers out there will be acutely familiar with this scenario and one of the reasons that I am now telling my story is for you to know that giving up is not an option if the system is to change for the better. I still have flashbacks whenever a doctor or health worker is in the news claiming they raised concerns but were met with silence or even worse with false accusations, and/or dismissal. A study on the emotional sequelae of whistleblowing in nurses by Peters et al[19] documented the impact on the emotional health of all involved in whistleblowing events and, furthermore, highlighted the intensity of emotional symptoms suffered by participants as well as the extended duration of time these symptoms. They also concluded that symptoms of anxiety, depression, hypervigilance and flashbacks were commonplace and are consistent with definitions of post-traumatic stress disorder and more serious outcomes including suicide[20-23].

It is disheartening to hear of the inevitable enquiry into the next health scandal (the latest is Lucy Letby where Dr Ravi Jayaram raised concerns about Letby to management at the Countess of Chester Hospital). Little has changed (*See a conflicted Jax Teller, page 23*). The recommendations of the Bristol inquiry have not been acted upon sufficiently to change the culture of the NHS. Mr Mayhem and the gavel came down again at the Reaper's Table. I learned much later, after I was sacked that the management team was awarded on the back of waiting list fiddles (although the Taylor Report did not criticise individuals in the management team). Michelle Masson made a statement for the Employment Tribunal (ET Case no. 1400692/2003). She worked at the Trust from 1992 initially personal administrator, moving up to become waiting list co-ordinator. The reason she left the Trust was because she made protected disclosures about the waiting list figures. The BBC took up the story and the Taylor report followed. Following my appointment she was aware in 1993, funding for a second cardiologist was being sought. The Trust had problems in meeting targets in cardiology and Dr Wakely was reluctant to do additional work because he was pushing for a second cardiologist appointment. Michelle reported that bullying and harassment is endemic in the Trust. In March 2000, she was told to remove 120 out-patients from the waiting list by two managers. In early 2002, the outpatient manager told her that "Dr Forbat was not doing his job properly." At a meeting with managers, she was told the Trust were looking at ways of 'getting rid of him' (*Dr Forbat*), but they had to be careful. The comment was made by the medical director in a meeting attended by the outpatient manager. Michelle said she was well aware there was a lot of activity on behalf of the Trust management trying to gain evidence all the time. When she was the duty manager, I called her about the lack of junior cover on the wards and radiology cover for emergency pacing. My calls were witnessed by a manager staying with her at the time. Michelle kept meeting notes in workbooks. She had no doubt the Trust were gathering evidence to get rid of me. Her assumption here was because I was not hitting targets to get waiting lists down (*I had reduced clinic numbers to safe levels as there were only five-minute slots. However, I think she was unaware I was raising concerns over patient harm!*) and she said, "It is clear Dr Forbat was not going to take the matter lying down."

A few years later, after two further consultant appointments, the British Cardiovascular Society reviewed the cardiology services at Weston General and supported many of the concerns I raised. The cardiologist appointment following my sacking lasted only a year before he left for another job. Recruitment remained a problem for some time. The trust now employs three cardiologists headed by the consultant who was SpR in training at the BRI during my tenure at Weston and with sessions at the BRI.

Chapter 9

The Merry-go-Round 2002-2021

Dr David Drew: Consultant paediatrician at Walsall Manor Hospital June 21, 2006, Kyle Keen bruises noted but no follow-up action was taken and he was discharged. Serious case review in 2009. David Drew was sacked for gross misconduct and insubordination for failing to accept the panel's instructions and for disclosing confidential information in relation to other matters.

Dr Raj Mattu: Consultant cardiologist Walsgrave Hospital in Coventry, suspended 2002 then sacked in 2010, after warning that patients were dying because of cost-cutting practices introduced by the Trust, upheld unfair dismissal in April 2014.

Dr Kevin Beatt: Consultant cardiologist at Croydon University Hospital's department for interventional heart procedures from 2007 until he was fired in September 2012 following the death in 2011 of a patient when bosses had suspended his most senior nurse hours before he performed the surgery, leaving him without a nurse with even basic understanding of the procedure for 20 minutes. A tribunal in 2014 found no evidence of wrongdoing by Dr Beatt.

As a consequence of my sacking from Weston General Hospital, my debts accrued and I had to decide how to maintain the family without job security and loss of my private practice income. If I took another NHS post, I would have to declare bankruptcy. I decided to continue working as a locum consultant and became an '*agency*' doctor, effectively on zero-hours contracts.

I was free to seek employment as a locum a couple of months after the NCAA report. I was working away from family in a six-week locum in a small Trust in Manchester and have vivid memories contemplating my future career as a doctor, whilst sitting alone in a restaurant on the evening of my birthday! I messaged my friends and spoke with my family in the subdued lighting of the restaurant as I dined alone and imagined a birthday cake with candles alight, but I couldn't extinguish them or the feeling of abandonment by the NHS and everything I had worked so hard for.

Fortunately, a few weeks later, I secured a locum at Walsgrave Hospital Coventry lasting 18 months. I was replacing Dr Raj Mattu's role since he was on "garden leave" (suspended) under investigation by the Trust following his whistleblowing. I had the advantage of knowing the consultants there, one of them on the appointment committee at West Cumberland.

My situation until March 2024, has been 24 years as career locum. I have worked in over 31 Trusts all around the UK, throughout England, Scotland, Wales and even the Isle of Man. The widespread shortage of consultants with over 10% of unfilled posts makes long-term agency work possible but not without its problems. Trusts when desperate pay agency rates as NHS locum rates are unattractive when paid at 50% of the consultant scale whatever the seniority of the doctor. However, since IR35 tax rules have been imposed on locums, net income has gone down. (See Episode 6 "AK-51", page 194).

In my experience there are major issues in the organisation leading to problems with retention and subsequent recruitment of a suitable replacement. It is unusual to find a long-term locum in a well-run department wanting to expand, as they are more likely to appoint 'in-house', promoting trainees (as with Weston, after I and a second consultant moved on). There are always issues in any Trust between some departments or individuals causing friction and if significant, often leading to dysfunction in the unit. This may be the in form of personality clashes, bullying, jealousy, protectionism of private income and departmental rivalry. When accepting a locum, one is unaware of the dynamics until in the post and navigating this can be a challenge. One stands out simply by being 'the locum' and if your clinical practice is different from their accepted norms, it can be seen as 'wrong' even if it is accepted normal practice in your substantive post or other locums. You can be seen as an asset to the department, relieving pressure on the workload, yet at the same time as a threat to an individual. You just don't know who the conductor is or who is playing which tune, and this can be stressful. Add in the interaction with managers and various staff, it often becomes impossible to know how to meet expectations or who to trust if you have any concerns regarding patient care. Raising any concerns is expected of all of us with the duty of candour, however, it is another area of trepidation. It is a great advantage if you know a colleague in the department or the Trust from your training years or previous jobs as they can vouch for you. It is common in hospitals to have staff that have not worked outside their local hospital environment and are unaware there are different practices to their own, or the 'correct way' to do things. This can be true in a small hospital or a tertiary centre. Rarely is anyone going to tell you the local *modus operandum* and they won't know your experience. Locums are therefore vulnerable to unfair criticism and complaints. In a locum a decade later at Pilgrim Hospital Boston, Lincolnshire, I was approached on coronary care on my second day by the new clinical lead, a diabetologist, who had just become medical director who remembered me from West Cumberland Hospital in Whitehaven, when he was a junior in the diabetes firm. He said there were major problems in the cardiology department and as Lincoln led on this since reconfiguration after the CQC report, there was no clear leadership locally and he wanted my advice. He asked to discuss the problems with me, and we agreed to a meeting later that week. This was not totally unexpected as, before taking up this locum, I was aware that the hospital remained in special measures after the Keogh review. However, prior to accepting the post I was reassured by a colleague who was the regional cardiology lead in Lincoln County, that there were no issues of higher mortality now and the reason for special measures continuing was related to the need for integration of services of three trusts, Grantham, Boston and Lincoln.

I saw the cardiologist from Lincoln when visiting in Pilgrim Hospital on a Monday morning, when he was there for a clinic and discussed pacing, angiography and ward rounds. I showed him my heart failure diuretic planner, which he said could be used. I was scheduled to have an induction morning and start with clinics, TOE and pacing sessions then rotate to coronary care as the cardiologist of the week in November. I was employed on a three-month contract as one of four consultants, but two were absent on leave and the remaining one who was meant to be there when I started was also absent. I soon became aware of several problems. Initially, I found that there were delays in echo reports and no images available at the CCU terminals, so I had to review them in the cardiology department several floors below. Cardiac physiologists also overruled requests from locum consultants! I needed to see the echos on the patients I had seen the two days before, to decide on management as all patients needed a consultant cardiologist's review. I let the ward know and arrived on the ward at 10.45 and Sister was agitated because I was not there at 09.30. Two patients in ITU required an urgent echo. There was no technician one afternoon, so I saw the patients and did their echos after my round. I soon came across a patient who had complications with the diagnosis of prosthetic valve endocarditis (infection of an artificial heart valve) following his discharge. He was sent home after requests for crucial diagnostic tests called a transthoracic (TTE) and transoesophgeal echo (TOE) were not done. Consequently, the diagnosis was missed, and he went home without treatment. This patient had a stroke due to the infection growing on the aortic valve breaking off and going to the brain and a subsequent TOE revealed a damaged aortic valve and an aortic root abscess. The patient needed urgent surgery for heart failure due to a leaking infected valve. I referred him for redo surgery to a surgeon I had worked with at Glenfield Regional Cardiothoracic Centre where he had an uneventful operation and fortunately the long-term outcome was good.

It was only a week later that I was joined by the cardiologist due to be in Pilgrim Hospital to greet me and show me the department, but I had still had no formal induction to the service. I joined the pacemaker list in the expectation of returning to pacing, as I have years of experience but 'with a significant break'. I was expected to buddy with a colleague until seen to be up to speed. I watched as the pacemaker implant went smoothly but at the end, the instruments, needles (sharps) and swabs on the operating trolley were about to be removed by the scrub nurse into the waste bins and I asked if they had been counted. The cardiologist said, 'We do not count instruments here' and I was shocked as this is normal practice to make sure nothing is left in or on the patient unaccounted for or caught in the various drapes that could cause injury. A needle stick injury might transmit infection such as hepatitis. There was not a 'WHO' (World Health Organisation) checklist for surgery before the start of an operating list for safety as I expected, or another debrief after, this aimed at reducing errors. Everyone involved should be introduced at the start of the session and know their roles and the lists reviewed, thus giving the opportunity for members of the team to raise any concerns, such as whether all necessary equipment is available, whether recent problems with it are resolved, or that all appropriate staff present. Each patient is then checked in against a standard checklist. At the end there is usually another checklist and debrief with the opportunity for any concerns to be raised, state what was done well (such as dealing with complications of a case) and what could be done better (e.g. reduced delays in collecting patients from the wards, ensuring patient consent was done the day before) next time.

I continued with the locum but after ten days I was told I was no longer needed! On Monday evening 27.10.14 I received an e-mail from my agency saying my contract was ending that Friday, only four days' notice from Tuesday, yet I had agreed to two weeks' notice with the agency. No clinical issues were given. I rang the medical director for more information and he said it was a result of complaints about my late ward round, the way I worked was 'not what they wanted', he warned me "***not to dig deeper and just leave***". I believe he too was afraid of meeting Mr Mayhem. On Tuesday morning following the Monday evening e-mail terminating my locum I rang colleague in Lincoln, and he said he had no idea that this had occurred! He said it should have been raised with him. He said he would investigate and get back. However, I have not had any contact feedback since. The only conclusion I come to is the Trust (The Lincoln Charter) management was keeping things 'in house', a common strategy, so the reputation of the Charter is protected.

A routine inspection of the Pilgrim Hospital was made on 1 and 2 May 2014 as part of the wider inspection of United Lincolnshire Hospitals NHS Trust (https://www.cqc.org.uk/location/RWDLA/reports). The hospital was last inspected on 1-2 July 2014. The trust was chosen for inspections because it was an example of a 'high risk' trust. Sir Bruce Keogh's review (Keogh Mortality Review) in 2013 found significant concerns and the trust was placed in 'special measures' as a result[25]. I had made a record of over 20 incidents, in my short stay.

The hospital was rated as requiring improvement. Core services for accident and emergency (A&E), medical care, surgery and maternity were found, overall, to require improvement.

The previous year it was inspected on 21, 25 June and 2, 4, 5 July 2013 when the Care Quality Commission was contacted by the Bruce Keogh Rapid Response Team, as they had concerns about the staffing levels at the hospital, particularly at night and weekends. The CQC undertook three unannounced inspections to the hospital, one on a Friday night. Staff were not confident in the reporting system and told us that feedback was inconsistent between managers. One doctor said, "I don't think anything is being fed up to the Board. We occasionally and perhaps get an email from the medical directorate about an incident telling us not to do something."

Since the contract had been terminated for my locum, I wrote on 29th October 2014 to the CQC, with a summary of my concerns. This was in my opinion a protected disclosure, sent strictly in confidence. I subsequently learned the pacing service was paused, whilst changes were introduced (I imagine, including the WHO checklist) and some staff retraining. I also learned the commissioners for the cardiology service had been given the report by the CQC to act on it and they forwarded my confidential letter in entirety to the regional centre linked to the Trust! I was afraid now I would be known as a whistleblower, and seen to be a problem in the whole county and this could impact any chance of further work should I want it in the region. The CQC later wrote and apologised. Indeed, as a result of my experience, I would not feel safe going back there to work. The Charters thus closed ranks after having made changes demanded by the CQC. They avoided publicity to protect the reputation of the local unit and the regional centre overseeing them.

The CD for medicine at Boston has since moved Trusts and has provided me with his honest recollections, albeit over a decade ago.

"I was CD for medicine at Boston, but cardiology was more pan-trust and run by its director, well thought of in the trust and most importantly had the eyes and ears of Medical director/CEO etc. This was the time when there were pensionable clinical excellence points to boost salary, which possibly a group could get due to activities etc.

The Boston issue was primarily due to difficulties in recruiting cardiology consultants to Boston and maintaining a viable rota. Due to the difficulties, I think it was decided interventional cardiology to be firmly established on Lincoln site and there were lot of discussions regarding door to balloon time etc. We would have had 2 site cardiology if we could have recruited adequate number of consultants in cardiology, but unfortunately we struggled, mostly from Europe and they didn't have dual CCT, which created another problem. Many consultants in Boston were aggrieved and kept saying services are being stripped from Boston to Lincoln ...but that is only because of Boston's inability to recruit, ballooning trust deficit due to locum pay, patient safety issues etc.

This gives a perspective from my end. I wasn't aware about any pacing set issue and I couldn't remember you being suspended. I just presumed you left because Boston was not up to the mark. The place had lots of Locums anyway."

(See Episode 7, "Old Bones", page 194).

As a locum there, bullying was not initially apparent, but I was approached by a cardiac physiologist (technician) after one pacing session when I was under considerable pressure during my list and told about bullying in the department. The first patient on my list for pacemaker implants was sent without ECG information in the records. I required sight of this to go ahead, since without this there was no indication for me to implant the pacemaker. I had to contact the referring cardiologist who was only available by phone and I delayed starting, waiting for a reply from him to confirm if there was evidence not seen by me but with him, indicating the need for pacing before I went ahead and implanted the pacemaker. I was promised the traces after the procedure, but when these materialised and after reviewing the traces, I was not convinced of a strong indication for pacing. A second case followed later where the patient did not need a pacemaker at all! The patient was added to my list after the list had been circulated, as a 'last-minute case' and a patient I had seen on the ward earlier that I had put next on the list was cancelled. This patient added had been transferred in the morning from another hospital before a prearranged referral for cancer surgery at a third hospital. This transfer followed a call to the senior consultant from a consultant anaesthetist at a pre-admission clinic in another hospital. The anaesthetist was concerned about surgery going ahead because he believed the patient had heart block (abnormal conduction on the ECG) that would make surgery unsafe without a pacemaker. The advice of a cardiologist at my Trust was to send the patient here for monitoring, i.e., observation. However, the admitting team believed incorrectly that the cardiologist transferred the patient with the intention for implantation of a permanent pacemaker implant, and so they were added to my list. The patient was brought straight from the ward and into the lab, as it was during COVID-19 and inpatients were not allowed to mix in the area with patients in the day case admitting area immediately outside the lab. The patient was brought through in a wheelchair and when I asked the patient what she understood about having a pacemaker and if she understood why it was needed, it seemed to me that she was confused and had not been told why or what was involved. Although a signature for consent for a pacemaker was obtained, I was concerned that this was not 'informed' consent. I reviewed her admission ECG in the notes, and it was normal. I told the staff I needed to see the evidence, but the consultant who accepted this patient was doing another procedure in the regional centre. I was then harassed by lab staff to get the patient 'on the table' and 'get on with the pacemaker' as the patient 'was getting cold' and was 'anxious'. I refused to do this and explained that there was no evidence to implant a pacemaker. I rang the other hospital and after a significant delay the cardiologist rang me back. He confirmed it was not his instruction to implant a pacemaker but to monitor the patient's rhythm. I sent the patient back to the ward distressed, aware she would miss her transport to the third hospital for her cancer treatment scheduled the following day. When she realised she did not need the pacemaker, she became even more upset. I felt vindicated and at the same time mentally exhausted having stood my ground and made the right decision in a hostile environment. There was also a locum cardiac physiologist working with me on this operation list and he came to me afterwards and thanked me for my actions. Similarly, the head of the department praised me and informed me about the bullying they had all endured. This was totally unacceptable and at the weekly cardiology consultant meeting I raised my concerns. Sadly, this is often encountered when a locum and not the only time I have been subject to harassment and unprofessional treatment in a catheter-lab setting.

A week later the consultant contacted me to say he had received a copy of the ECG the anaesthetist had been concerned about and revealed to me it was for another patient, not from the patient I was expected to implant the pacemaker! Before starting this locum, my agency had confirmed my contract was due to be extended at the end of the month for another three months into the New Year. However, a week later the agency said they no longer required my services. I took advice following the concerns raised by me and other staff and asked for a statement from a technician about their experience of bullying. However, they were not willing to put their name to a statement, perhaps fearing losing their job. The next revelation came the week after I had left: the CQC were due to inspect the Trust in the New Year! A locum who would raise concerns, as I had at the consultant weekly meeting, was not going to be welcome on-site during the CQC inspection and so by terminating my locum contract, the Charter had called on Mr Mayhem to defend their reputation. Colchester Hospital was featured on the ITV Tonight programme, *After Lucy Letby: Silence on the Wards* (20:30, 09 September 2023) and Nick Hulme who was *appointed* chief executive of Ipswich *Hospital* NHS Trust in January 2013 (now chief executive of Suffolk and Essex) was the only CEO agreeing to be interviewed on this programme. It was reported he feared unacceptable care is becoming the acceptable, stating " … a serious incident happens every day in a lot of hospitals up and down the country, my concern is because it has almost become business as usual we have become a bit, almost a bit anaesthetised to it." I don't know if he was aware of concerns that I raised in cardiology as I was sacked from the locum and I doubt the CQC were made aware when they did a follow-up visit in 2021.

CQC inspection of Colchester Hospital 2019:

Overall rating given was "Requires Improvement." The CQC found that the hospital provided safe, effective, and caring services, but that there were areas where improvements were needed. The hospital was rated as "Requires Improvement" in the categories of safety, responsiveness, and well-led.

Patient expectations are different and can also be influenced by local practices. Once confidence in a locum is undermined, especially if not supported by a colleague who knows them, the most likely outcome is the locum decides to leave, or it comes to an end by early termination or not extending the contract (these are typically three-month rolling contracts with a week's notice) as advertised. This is the 'merry-go-round' life of a locum. Complaints from patients are not uncommon in a career and are dealt with via PALS, where the doctor can respond and resolve any issues, usually a consequence of miscommunication. This is often not possible for a locum to deal with as delays mean the complaint does not materialise during the locum contract or, if it does, it may not be communicated to them and so dealt with by another consultant.

I held three locums before my first substantive post at a time when fewer suitable new consultant posts were forthcoming. These were all enjoyable. In the subsequent 29, 13 (45%) were a positive experience, 5 (13%) mixed experience and 11 (38%) part or all were a negative experience. Of the latter several stand out, three were terrible, six tolerable and two mixed, in that they went well until unexpected turns of events soured the experience near the end. (See Episode 8, "The Pull", see page 194.)

Previously, working was rewarding, until I realised most of the time conversations were going on behind my back. My impact on the individuals was being discussed by a few who

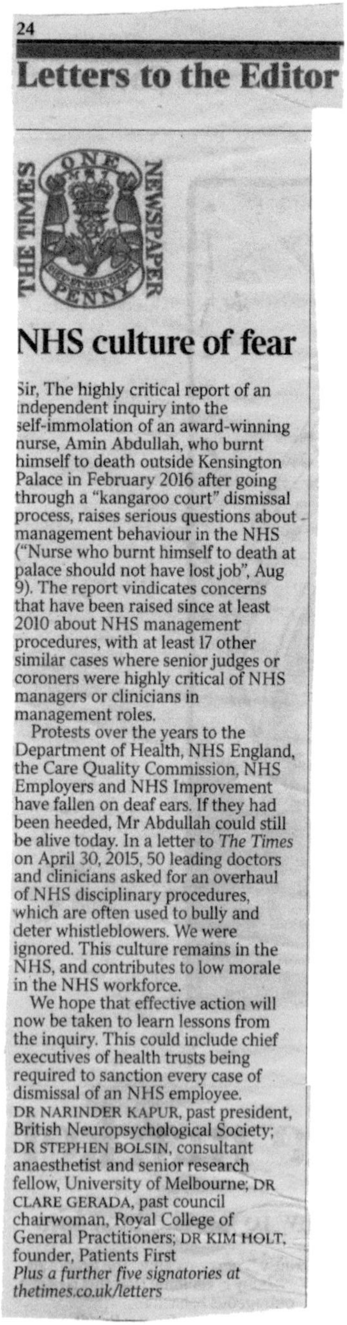
24

Letters to the Editor

THE TIMES ONE PENNY NEWSPAPER

NHS culture of fear

Sir, The highly critical report of an independent inquiry into the self-immolation of an award-winning nurse, Amin Abdullah, who burnt himself to death outside Kensington Palace in February 2016 after going through a "kangaroo court" dismissal process, raises serious questions about management behaviour in the NHS ("Nurse who burnt himself to death at palace should not have lost job", Aug 9). The report vindicates concerns that have been raised since at least 2010 about NHS management procedures, with at least 17 other similar cases where senior judges or coroners were highly critical of NHS managers or clinicians in management roles.

Protests over the years to the Department of Health, NHS England, the Care Quality Commission, NHS Employers and NHS Improvement have fallen on deaf ears. If they had been heeded, Mr Abdullah could still be alive today. In a letter to *The Times* on April 30, 2015, 50 leading doctors and clinicians asked for an overhaul of NHS disciplinary procedures, which are often used to bully and deter whistleblowers. We were ignored. This culture remains in the NHS, and contributes to low morale in the NHS workforce.

We hope that effective action will now be taken to learn lessons from the inquiry. This could include chief executives of health trusts being required to sanction every case of dismissal of an NHS employee.

DR NARINDER KAPUR, past president, British Neuropsychological Society; DR STEPHEN BOLSIN, consultant anaesthetist and senior research fellow, University of Melbourne; DR CLARE GERADA, past council chairwoman, Royal College of General Practitioners; DR KIM HOLT, founder, Patients First

Plus a further five signatories at thetimes.co.uk/letters

felt exposed or threatened by a confident locum inadvertently exposing poor or unusual local practice (I was exposed to wide variations across different hospitals around the UK) by his own actions, challenging them outside comfort zones. The team structure and its function were compromised, discipline was lost, staff morale deteriorated and I believe the quality of patient care had definitely suffered.

In each Trust where I had a bad experience, I found personalities that mirrored characters in the cast of *Sons of Anarchy*. This included individuals in my substantive posts who had undue influence in the organisation and on me as an individual. They reflect the culture in the hospitals concerned. These observations may not be new to those working in the NHS and other large organisations. However, I have not met or know of any other consultants with my level of exposure working in so many departments, over a prolonged period of their career and I am only aware of a handful who were prepared to stand up to these challenges. Before accepting a locum, I always search for reports by the CQC for advanced knowledge. Invariably, these reports do not get to the heart of these problems, rarely scratching below the surface of what is carefully presented to the CQC during scheduled visits.

Only after investigations in the form of inquiries, such as the Francis Report following Stafford, do the underlying issues get aired in public. They included a culture of fear, lack of leadership, lack of accountability and neglect of dignity. I have witnessed this repeatedly and when appropriate I have raised concerns. I was one of 290 whistleblowers who testified (164 oral, 87 written statements, 39 provisional statements) to Sir Robert Francis. (Episode 9, "Hell Followed", see page 194).

Chapter 10

Family Matters – Life Outside Medicine

As a newly married pre-registration house officer in 1980, I remained a 'junior doctor' through senior house officer posts, registrar posts until 1993, when I was a locum consultant. The work as a newly qualified doctor was intense, commonly the on-call rota was alternate nights and weekends (one-in-two rotas) meaning one had to be resident in the hospital 120 hours a week. When I was in my first six months post-registration house job in the renal unit, my wife would join me in the on-call room at St Thomas's, bringing her portable black and white TV and snacks. When at night and on call, she would be sidling up to me as we shared a single bed with a dubious quality hospital mattress and invariably when we managed to get comfortable, my bleep would go off! My wife had sleep deprivation alongside mine! Moving between hospitals in London meant we could remain in our first flat as our family grew until we had to move to Leicester with our two daughters to take up my training post in cardiology. The on-call was less frequent but days remained long.

Holidays were spent in a time-share in Fureguola Spain each summer. I had little time for hobbies or sport until we moved to Cumbria when I took up dinghy sailing on Bassenthwaite Lake.

After I was sacked and after I returned to work in February 2003, I decided to take up locum consultant posts in cardiology anywhere I could in the UK, in order to avoid bankruptcy, so we kept our house and maintained the children at their school. This meant I was not at home during the week and away many weekends for much of my last 22 years, until March 2024. My time away from home during the week was divided between working during the day and passing the time in my evenings shopping for essentials, cooking if facilities were available or eating out if not. In some locations I regularly went to the cinema to watch the latest films. Whenever the occasion arose for a job with a nearby relative, I would visit. I rang home daily as there were no smartphones in the early years, so no Facetime to see the children. Long journeys home for the weekend break began by packing up my laundry for my wife to wash and replenish my wardrobe for the following week. If I was commuting daily, it could be up to 2½ hours each way so almost half a day travelling. I was burning the candle at both ends and after an evening meal I was less useful than I would have wanted, collapsing on the settee in front of the TV. Meanwhile the children were doing well at school, which was rewarding considering the financial commitment and the infrequent input from my side. My wife was driving around 1000 miles a week on the school runs as one daughter was in the Modern Pentathlon squad at Millfield. This required morning and evening swimming training before and after normal school times with running, fencing, shooting and horse riding somewhere in the mix. My wife made an early run to drop off our budding athlete (selected for the Olympic Start programme), then returned to collect the other two, repeating this double run twice after school finished.

We live in an old stone-built property with metal Crittall windows in wooden frames and we have a garden with split-level lawns due to the underlying Mendip rock formation, with woodland surrounds forever encroaching inwards. This required regular maintenance by me as we could not afford to pay for a workman or gardener. Fortunately, my wife has green fingers, and I was left the task of mowing the grass, trimming trees and felling those fallen or dead ones for logs to use in our wood burners. We have three mature apple trees that provide a large crop each year and I pressed these to make fresh juice and an occasional batch of cider. These apples were not suitable for eating but the juice extracted was delicious and they make the best baked apples ever.

When I belonged to Bassenthwaite Sailing Club in Cumbria I sailed a second-hand wooden Mirror dinghy bought off the haematologist. This came with us when moving to Bristol and I joined Chew Valley Lake Sailing Club. Here I added to my fleet with a second-hand Lazer 13, much larger for the family. Only my youngest daughter took any interest. On one very windy weekend we went fully reefed down, out onto the lake by which time the water was whipping up a choppy swell. I will never forget when we capsized (not the only ones here!) and were unable to get back in. I was holding onto the successfully re-righted Lazer with one hand and the rear of my daughter's life jacket with the other hand when she piped up with, "*Nice knowing you dad!*" thinking the end was coming! We of course were quickly picked up by the rescue boat and brought ashore, dried off and had a hot drink. We visited local farm parks and rarely went on long walks despite Mendips on our doorstep.

Annual holidays became sparse and except for visiting my eldest daughter twice in ten years after she emigrated to Sydney, Australia. I worked until any locum ended and took breaks only when I had no work. There is no guarantee or security of income, so making savings was essential while income was there to tide one through the dry times. There is no holiday pay, sick pay (as when I was ill and quarantined with COVID-19) or paid study leave as a locum. The contract states 'included' in the hourly rates. This is a real farce as most are short contracts that won't cover anything, so I self-financed these breaks between jobs in order to survive! We had to switch from a repayment to an interest-only mortgage on our new home soon after and this had the advantage of a chequebook facility to use against the equity in our house. When my mortgage is up in three years we will not own it, unless a miraculous source of income comes my way! All I can hope for any equity left will enable us to downsize. This is the consequence of being a whistleblower. There are rarely means of obtaining any realistic and adequate compensation whether through the courts or tribunals. These avenues are not suitable vehicles and are definitely not fit for purpose for a whistleblower, especially for me, as I was sacked so the Trust (Charter) could avoid a tribunal and all the negative publicity that would follow.

As a peripatetic locum I missed much of the time a father would expect to spend with his children as they grew up, lost years of precious time when normally family would be together with my wife and consequently the day-to-day burden of running the family fell mainly on her. Many doctors in my situation never return to any work, often suffering depression and some take their own lives[18]. There is no support financially and no reconciliation with the Trusts or compensation for disruption of careers, lost income (including pension) and long-lasting reputational damage.

I have made a calculation based on the fact that over the last 20 years, several hundred doctors have found themselves in this position and using the settlement figure for Dr Raj Mattu of 2.5 million pounds, the Government should have a fund of two to three billion pounds to compensate everyone affected. I am advised this was an exceptional settlement figure. However, there may be many more whistleblowers than I estimate here as there is no database. Another includes Kevin Beatt cardiologist, who was awarded

8 2GM Monday February 9 2015 | THE TIMES

News

Jail for NHS bosses who lie about poor care in hospitals

Chris Smyth Health Editor

NHS bosses face two years in jail for lying about poor care, as ministers intensify a campaign against a culture of cover-up in the health service.

Hospitals that cannot prove they have owned up and apologised to patients for mistakes will also be fined £10,000 for losing negligence claims under plans to be announced today.

Jeremy Hunt, the health secretary, said that the move "sends a strong message that covering up mistakes will not be tolerated".

On Wednesday Sir Robert Francis, QC, who led an inquiry into the neglect of hundreds of patients at Stafford Hospital, will make recommendations on how to encourage staff to speak out.

The government is creating a new "false or misleading information offence", which will make it a crime to knowingly give incorrect data to regulators or official audits.

Hospitals face unlimited fines if they are convicted as organisations and could also be publicly shamed by being forced to tell patients or display posters about their lies. Senior staff who "consented or connived" in the deception could be fined or imprisoned for up to two years.

The offence will apply to any information that hospitals are legally required to publish or submit to official bodies and is aimed at chief executives and senior medical staff. Ministers concede that it is likely to be used rarely, but the measure was condemned by doctors' leaders, who said that it could make staff too scared to speak up.

Since the end of last year NHS organisations have had a legal duty to admit mistakes to patients and the latest plans aim to penalise those that do not.

Hospitals that cannot prove they have been fully open when facing a negligence claim will have to reimburse £10,000 to the NHS Litigation Authority, which pays out claims.

Peter Walsh, from the charity Action against Medical Accidents, praised the plans, which he said could have held bosses at Stafford accountable. "It sends a clear message that this is socially important and we don't want to see this sort of behaviour," he said.

However, Mark Porter, chairman of the British Medical Association's governing council, said that introducing a criminal law could diminish doctors' confidence about raising concerns.

"We need a culture of openness within the NHS, not where speaking up can leave doctors feeling harassed or facing punitive action," he said.

Mr Walsh dismissed notions that such a law could deter staff from coming forward. "It's such a fundamental thing. If a doctor is prepared to lie or cover up, they are not fit to be a doctor. You don't mess around and say 'We have to turn a blind eye' as we've done for decades because of some vague notion of blame culture," he said.

Figures published yesterday suggest that there are improving death rates at eight out of 11 hospitals put into "special measures" after the Stafford scandal because of concerns over poor care.

Dr Foster, the consultancy which analysed the changes made, said that this was significantly different from the rest of the country and was unlikely to be down to chance.

Leading article, page 28

£870,000 in compensation from Croydon Health Services NHS trust, which sacked him after he raised safety concerns after a patient's death. A similar total could be arrived at by many smaller awards. Critically, there should be accountability for the leaders in these Trusts making certain that they are not recycled into other posts. If there is clear evidence that they have overseen patient harm and suppressed the truth, they should be prosecuted and, if found guilty, fined or be considered for a custodial sentence.

At the time of writing, the Thirlwall Inquiry into the Countess of Chester Hospital is expected to report in Autumn 2025. Let us hope by the time this book is read the reaction to the Lucy Letby enquiry and any others since will at last start the healing of our NHS. Since her conviction, there is an appeal for a retrial.

My private practice income was sparse and when I had to liquidate my company, HMRC lifted the protection of a Ltd company status and claimed back my unpaid director's loan. The only way I could pay my tax arrears was by agreement with HMRC for a settlement, in turn forcing me to transfer my NHS Pension to a private one and use the 25% tax-free sum that I qualified for after 55 years old, to pay my debts. Furthermore, I was missing out on a lump sum on retirement, had I remained employed in the NHS. From then on, no new cars to look forward to and since then I have continued to do my own car repairs and services. My 2001 330Ci BMW racked up 720,000 miles with two gearbox reconditions, first after 350,000 and one engine replacement with a second-hand engine after BMW failed to sort out a blocked radiator, overheating the aluminium block ruining the engine. BMW settled out of court.

I regularly commuted to Glasgow on day trips to the Nuffield clinic where I had a dwindling private practice and this helped me survive between locums. I would regularly stop off at Lancaster Services for a bacon roll and coffee, then again at Lesmahagow, 20 miles south of Glasgow where my friend Derek Palmer owns a garage and serviced my BMW when I was out of my depth. He is a motorsport expert and winner of Grand Tour racing in Nissan race-tuned cars, also an innovator who launched his team 'Speed Scotland' who are attempting and yet to beat 300mph the land speed record for naturally aspirated cars with 'The Flower of Scotland', a bullet-shaped car. We first met up at Glasgow airport departure lounge on one of my Thursday evening trips home to Bristol on Easyjet. Standing next to each other in a queue and as unknown friends-to-be at that time, were musing at a gaggle of ladies in pink attire with tinsled hair and t-shirts emblazoned with slogans depicting a hen night out. I think I started up a conversation about the scene in the queue as it was snaking ahead of us towards the security check-in. We soon found we had common interests in cars, aviation and boats. Derek was going to spend a weekend on his canal boat in Somerset. We talked about my father's career in aviation as an aeronautical engineer, his origins as an evacuee from Budapest Hungary, his role in Vickers at Brooklands, Weybridge and flying in Canberras with the first fly-by-wire missile tests for the MOD. On cars, Derek was a mine of information, and he offered to help out with my BMW servicing, as it was still running in (at about 200,000 miles!). I learned a great deal over the years, and it put me in good stead for future car repairs I have had to do to save on BMW's expensive services.

I wrote to Derek on 26 June, 2025.

> *"Derek, I reviewed my CV and realise we have been friends over 25 years now! Would you consider writing something about me from your knowledge and perspective?"*

Derek has dyslexia, important to mention here (Derek is happy about me stating this) because he had to make a real effort during his busy schedule, to compose his thoughts and get them down in a word document. His achievements surpass any issue that might be from dyslexia, as he has excelled in motorsport, including his attempts (almost succeeding) in making the 300mph land speed record for a normally aspirated engine in the car he designed and built, 'Speed Scotland', that can be found online.

I wrote again on 24 August:

> "*Anyway, just some thoughts came to me while relaxing between renovations on my e46 and VW repairs for the MOT. Some philosophical thoughts for*

you! I thought about friendship. Since I am without a brother or father and only recently gained a son-in-law, I realised male friends are vital and indeed our friendship is one of the longest I have had, second only to another from medical school. Rarely meeting but always in touch. Both with same outlook and sense of humour. For me it is great to know that someone of a completely different background can have similar interests and wondered what it means to you, especially as I have asked you to write a piece for my memoir. I suppose I will find out soon enough. Enjoy the weekend with family."

Derek's contribution arrived at last in my e-mail on 17 October:

"I first met Lance on a flight to Bristol. He was commuting home after working in Glasgow, and I was heading south to my narrowboat. By chance, we ended up on the same flight most weeks—him heading home, me either bound for the boat or off to a race circuit for work.

It was one of those fortunate coincidences. Lance loved cars, and I make my living restoring and preparing racing cars, so we were never short of things to talk about.

Over the years Lance had obviously decided one of the ways to save the planet was not to constantly renew his cars, he did a huge mileage and loved driving his BMW 330 Coupe even when others would have decided it was too old.

He managed to get almost three-quarters of a million miles out this car before it was damaged in an accident and what happened? We scoured the country to find one exactly the same to replace it and the old one was kept for parts. In the process we probably ventured into areas never envisaged by BMW as far as durability was concerned.

From my side, I found him absolutely fascinating—not only a skilled heart surgeon, but with a family history that's every bit as remarkable as he is.

Over the years of our friendship, we've shared plenty of knowledge, and I can honestly say I've learned a great deal from him. Lance had a telemedicine system up and running almost as soon as the internet could support it, and he's helped my family and me countless times with advice and support from miles away—something for which I'll always be grateful. I like to think that, in return, I've been able to help him a little with his own passions—his cars.

On one visit to the Brooklands Museum, I noticed that the person responsible for the display of Britain's groundbreaking missile programme shared Lance's surname. As it turned out, that was no coincidence—his father had been one of the main figures behind it.

As you read this book, you'll be reading the story of one of the most honest and intelligent people I've ever had the privilege to know. Lance doesn't suffer fools, and his mind is as sharp as a razor. That sharpness has helped him solve some of the more unusual challenges I've faced over the years, and I've no doubt that his strong principles have, at times, brought their own challenges too.

I, for one, am looking forward to reading this book—and I'm certain it will make for an interesting and inspiring read.

Derek"

Sadly in 2019 one evening driving to a clinic on a poorly lit motorway I drifted, on reflection possibly a 'micro-sleep', and I hit some gravel. I lost steering control then glanced the central barrier and the car spun pirouetting a few times before stopping on the hard shoulder facing in my original direction of travel. No other cars were in the vicinity. My rear bumper and exhaust box were in the road, various parts of my rear lights were scattered around the motorway, and the front of the car was a mess. I was glad had recently cut out the rust and mig-welded my sills so the body of the car was intact. A few cars were arriving across the three lanes, stopping a few hundred short of me and watched as I collected bits of my car and carried them onto the hard shoulder. A very lucky escape; if I were of a religious nature I think I would believe my brother was looking over me on that day. I called the AA and while waiting a patrol car must have been alerted and stopped and checked I was ok. I hired a car until I found another younger model 330Ci, 2005 registration with 81,000 miles and with money my late brother Anthony (Ant' to me) promised before he died at only 63 years old. He knew I could not afford another. I bought this and exchanged the wooden gear knob for the tired leather one in the new car before the old car was scrapped. That gear knob has now travelled over a million miles!

I clocked over 238,000 miles, still servicing and repairing this later model. However, following pothole damage to the wheel and steering then a gearbox leak meant its time was up. I found my third iteration 330Ci with over 112,000 miles on the clock, and now a proud owner of the wooden gear knob. I have stripped the old one down to the metal shell for parts I keep as spares. Others, I am selling, hoping to recoup the cost of this car.

Ant and I were very close. We went to Cubs and then Sea Scouts together, cycling from our home in Surbiton for several miles. On return we would stop off, if we had sixpence left over from pocket money, and buy chips wrapped in newspaper and devour them as we cycled, finishing them shortly before arriving home for tea that mum had prepared for us, as if we had not eaten in a week! When we moved to Weybridge we continued to cycle to Ajax Sea Scouts in Thames Ditton, over seven miles and including a very steep hill from Hersham onto Esher. It was always a race to do the run in under 25 minutes. We had heavy metal framed bikes with stermi-archer gears (not lightweight versions with derailer gears – we could not afford these). Ant had straight handlebars whereas mine had drop handlebars and yet Ant, 14 months older, was stronger in his legs and would beat me up the steep hills with his upright posture, as I followed head down close behind peddling furiously!

My time in Ajax is summarised here by George Barber, who was the Ajax Scout leader at the time.

Lance Forbat

"I have known Lance since, as a boy of eleven years, he joined 4th Thames Ditton 'Ajax' Sea Scouts. I was Sea Scout Leader at the time. Lance was following a tradition in the Forbat family in that his older brother Tony had joined Ajax a year or so before him and their father John was a Sea Scout in Putney and later became Assistant County Commissioner for Water Activities in Surrey. During his time in the Sea Scout Troop Lance excelled at all the activities and was appointed patrol leader from fourteen to sixteen years of age. Lance led his patrol exceptionally well at camps and on the water including coxswain's cruises when a patrol would man a 20 foot gig and set off under oars on an adventure on tidal waters at places such as Poole Harbour, Chichester Harbour or the east coast rivers Crouch, Blackwater and Deben.

Preparation for these cruises led by the Patrol Leader included chartwork, selection of overnight camping gear, menu selection and safe storage of food, camp gear and personal gear in the boat. Once the boat crew shoved of at the beginning of the cruise they were on their own until they returned to base, usually a summer camp site, the next day. There were no mobile phones in the 1970s when Lance led his cruise. It was testament to the faith in Lance that the leaders had that he was allowed to be in charge of the cruise at the tender age of fifteen.

At the age of sixteen Lance moved up to the Venture Sea Scout Unit and was an enthusiastic member through to the age of twenty during which time he took part in the DoE Award programme, gaining bronze, silver and gold awards. For the gold award expedition he took a crew around Chichester and Langstone Harbours with the aim of collecting mud samples that were sent off for analysis to determine pollution levels.

At the age of twenty Lance became an Assistant Scout Leader when he was able to use all the experience gained in Ajax in the training of younger members. This he continued to do with breaks for university up until the time he moved away to practice medicine.

Since his early formative years and his time as a leader Lance has always maintained an interest in the progress of the Ajax Sea Scouts Group.

Written by George Barber

Trustee, 4th Thames Ditton "Ajax" Sea Scout Group "

Ant passed his 11 plus and passing the compulsory entrance exam, went to the prestigious Tiffin Grammar School in Kingston. He was exceptionally bright, particularly very good at maths. He went on to Emmanuel College Cambridge and in his first year achieved the highest mark in mathematics exams for Cambridge University! He loved rowing and earned an 'oar' in the Emmanuel College rowing eights. This, despite an uncorrected typo, was proudly hung on the wall of his living room. He married Jane, a solicitor, and had three sons. At around 62 years he went to his doctor feeling, mildly unwell after anaesthetic for a minor shoulder procedure. About a year later he thought he may have a gastric problem with bloating and went for investigation with an endoscopy and when reports came back normal, he had an abdominal ultrasound and set off for home. There was a terrible shock when he told us he was called back before getting home to be seen urgently for more tests. A rare cancer had taken over 95% of his liver! This non-endocrine pancreatic cancer typically produces no pain or other symptoms. He had intensive treatments over the next couple of years at the Marsden. Hopes were rising it was under control, but the cancer then stopped responding and he was given a short time to live. He had planned a one-week cruise on a Cunard liner and was now too unwell. His medical condition precluded any insurance if he had to cancel and typical of Ant, he generously offered the weeks to us. He knew we had not afforded a holiday in years. We had a brilliant time and had an excuse to 'dress up to the nines' each evening. A neighbouring couple of theirs had booked this cruise to join them and became new friends. On one lunchtime I was sitting near a table with one lady. She was having a loud telephone conversation I could not avoid overhearing. It sounded very medical, so I introduced myself. She was Victoria Townsend who, following the death of her son William, founded and ran a charity called Breatheon. The charity was set up to support parents of babies on ventilators with life-threatening illnesses, like her son William. I was subsequently persuaded to take on the role of medical director of her new charity of the same name for Long COVID-19 sufferers.

We returned after our cruise and Ant was in hospital, waiting for the latest scans and a treatment decision. He was sitting up smiling in his bed but my dearest, kindest big brother looked gaunt and yellow from jaundice. I could clearly see his liver was distorting his swollen abdomen, something no one ever wants to see, let alone in a loved one. (Four years on, writing this brought tears to my eyes.) Ant died peacefully at home on Tuesday 12 June, 2018, with family present having had excellent palliation in the last few weeks.

We saw less of our three sisters outside of the home. Yolande is the next below me and was into ballet and won a scholarship at Elmhurst. Dad could afford her fees more easily because he did not need to supplement my living costs at medical school, as I saved my vacation earnings working as a relief milkman for Job's Dairy. Yolande (Yo' to me – she doesn't like being called this now!) between professional work and establishing her successful ballet school, worked in interior design when injury brought her performance career to an end. Yolande continues to do exceptionally well, attaining more professional dancing qualifications as an examiner. She is married to Bob, and they have two daughters and recently a second granddaughter.

Wendy (Wendy Woo) my middle sister, was the quieter, more introverted one until she left home and blossomed in her own way, working in Boots and doing well. She did not have a regular partner and lived in a crowded rental apartment in London and in poor sanitary conditions. She did eventually get her own flat through the council and was very happy there. She never forgot a birthday and had presents in readiness for all her nephews and nieces. Sadly, Wendy developed breast cancer and living alone she hid it until it was too late, so it had spread widely, yet Wendy survived this until a flare-up of inflammatory bowel disease. It was not unusual for Wendy not to be in touch for a couple of days, but after the fourth day when she was uncontactable, the alarm was raised. Our family were spread around some distance away and we called the emergency services who discovered her lying dead in her flat. We believe she was lying on the floor for a few days before she was discovered. She was only 52 years old.

My youngest sister Sandra (known by friends as Sandy), seven years younger, was and remains 'bright as a button'. She eventually followed in my footsteps to study medicine at St. Thomas's and became consultant radiologist in northeast Scotland. She is now retired, two years before my writing this! She remains in Scotland with husband Al and with two daughters having left home, Sandra spends her days kayaking and with a house full of dogs (I have lost count how many) goes on long walks with them, occasionally joined by her daughters and Al. He is a Fast Jet pilot retired as Air Commodore, to Lossiemouth Royal Airforce. He flew Tornados and during the Iraq war was stationed in the USA and was unique as the only British fighter pilot who flew sorties in the 'stealth' bomber. He now enjoys his outdoor interests and charity work,

Life outside medicine was never totally divorced from the effects of my whistleblowing on the family dynamics. If a locum was short duration, or not extended as hoped, my wife would assume I caused some upset by speaking out or got frustrated or angry and there were arguments following which I knew however I protested, I could not win her over to my side. Such is the legacy of the trauma we experienced when I was suspended and then sacked from Weston. It is akin to coping with post-traumatic stress. Indeed, this is a common diagnosis after such life-changing events. It is just common practice the way that Trusts (the Charters) can hire and fire locums to meet their needs while minimizing the costs to their stretched finances. This is the life of anyone on 'zero hours' contracts. The advantage is the doctor can decide when and where he or she works but the employer also has this power at their disposal.

We have three daughters, the eldest qualified with a degree in fashion Journalism but the "Devil wore Prada" environment of the fashion industry didn't agree with her, so she emigrated to Australia, now living in Sydney and working as a buyer for Dinosaur Designs. She has two girls and unfortunately, due to the distance, we don't see them often enough other than on Facetime.

Our second daughter was a bundle of energy and joined Cockermouth swimming club, soon swimming in the top team and winning a swimming scholarship to Millfield School in Somerset. She boarded in the prep school and, soon noticed for her athleticism, she was enticed into joining the Millfield Modern Pentathlon team of five disciplines: swimming, shooting, running, riding and fencing. She was picked for the Olympic 'Start' programme. She later relinquished any Olympic hopes on entering the sixth form, having decided to concentrate on her A-levels and a vocational career. She is now married to Joe (ex-professional rugby union player at scrum half – prompting my return to the game of my teens, but only 'touch' rugby at 63 years!).

A late addition to our family of three girls, who is truly 'her own', by surprising us at her infant school concert, when she belted out 'Little Donkey' with a pure voice reminiscent of my mother at age six! She has no plans to follow this talent professionally, however, a rendition can occasionally slip out! A degree in English Literature and her wise decision, as not going to make it as a doctor, she has once more reinvented herself! First, she pursued a 'fitness fad', a podcast followed, then with a realisation that she could influence her peers, she developed a following and morphed from body image guru to personality promoter, inviting predominantly women to discuss their take on life in her blog 'Adulting'. She then decided to try her hand as an author, culminating with her first book, *Bad Influence: Reflections on a Life Lived Online*. No doubt by the time you read this, other fame may come her way!

It was important for my sanity, to maintain a work life balance while working as a locum away from home. I found a means of escapism in Glasgow during my longest locum, when I became a regular attender at the cinema. Subsequently, I was moving around the UK with shorter contracts and at 63 years of age, after watching Joe play for Wasps, I looked up local touch rugby clubs and paid £25.00 for a year membership to touch rugby at UWE Bristol. My wife had never seen me showing any interest in rugby when we had our children and thought it was a mid-life crisis, 60 being the new 'middle age' and my interest would not continue beyond the first year! Seven years on at the time of writing (70 on 3 March 2026), I can't imagine a week without an hour or two of this sport. I decided to write a book on my experience (*Touch Rugby and Physical and Mental Health – a Doctor's Experience, for publication in 2026)* and it includes a chapter with contributions from members of clubs I attended. This is one of my first contributions from Vaughan Rob from Canterbury Touch.

"Lance joined our touch rugby club in Canterbury in September 2021. Since then, Lance made a remarkable impact during his time with us, which sadly came to an end in October 2022. Despite this relatively short period, he left a lasting impression, embodying the spirit and vibrance that make this sport truly special. As a doctor, he not only shared his medical expertise but also a deep passion for promoting physical and mental wellbeing through active participation in sport. This was showed by his determination to attend sessions even after long shifts and poor weather.

Lance's commitment and dedication were evident in every training session. At an age when many might slow down, he played with the energy and enthusiasm of someone half his age, reminding us all that it's never too late to embrace a new challenge. His infectious positivity uplifted the team, creating a welcoming atmosphere where everyone felt valued, regardless of their skill level.

In our club, Lance seamlessly integrated into our community, forging friendships and fostering a sense of belonging. His experience resonates with the broader message of touch rugby: it is a sport that transcends age and background. As he often noted, anyone who is reasonably mobile—male or female—can participate and reap the physical and mental benefits that come from regular exercise.

From his perspective, the advantages of touch rugby extend far beyond the physical. It offers a unique social experience that encourages camaraderie and support, helping players improve their mental resilience and overall happiness. Lance's reflections emphasise how vital this sport can be for mental health, particularly in today's fast-paced world where stress can be overwhelming.'

Chapter 11

The GMC Challenge 2010, 2021-23

[Dr Raj Mattu: Consultant Cardiologist Walsgrave Hospital, in Coventry Suspended for eight years, then sacked in 2010, after warning that patients were dying because of cost-cutting practices introduced by Trust management, unfair dismissal in April 2014]

The GMC or the General Medical Council is a regulatory body in the United Kingdom responsible for overseeing the medical profession and maintaining the standards of medical practice. The General Medical Council plays a crucial role in ensuring the safety and well-being of patients and the public by setting and upholding the standards of medical education, training, and practice, in order to protect patients and improve medical education and practice across the UK.

In summary from GMC website:

1. Decide which doctors are qualified to work in the UK
2. Oversee UK medical education and training
3. Set the standards doctors need to follow throughout their careers
4. Where necessary, take action to prevent a doctor from putting the safety of patients, or the public's confidence in doctors, at risk.

Key roles and functions of the GMC are:

1. Licensing and Registration: The GMC is responsible for granting licenses to doctors, allowing them to practice medicine in the UK. It maintains a register of qualified medical practitioners, which is publicly accessible.
2. Medical Education and Training: The GMC sets the standards for undergraduate and postgraduate medical education and training

programs in the UK. It also approves medical schools and postgraduate training providers.
3. Professional Standards: The GMC defines and enforces the professional standards expected of doctors, including their behaviour, ethics, and conduct. This helps ensure that doctors provide high-quality care and maintain the trust of patients and the public.
4. Investigating Complaints: The GMC investigates complaints and concerns raised about doctors' conduct or fitness to practice. If necessary, it can take disciplinary action, such as issuing warnings, imposing conditions on a doctor's practice, or removing a doctor from the medical register.
5. Revalidation: The GMC introduced a system of revalidation, which requires doctors to demonstrate on an ongoing basis that they are up-to-date and fit to practice medicine.
6. Public Awareness and Advocacy: The GMC works to promote public awareness of healthcare.

Most doctors I know perceive the GMC not to be supportive of them or their professional status. There are several reasons. It is the result of the experience of many doctors in less published cases, where referrals are made in haste, or as vindictive or malicious referrals to punish or to silence outspoken doctors who are voicing any concerns and following GMP (good medical practice). There are also proven cases of increased referral to the GMC which is addressing discrimination, disadvantage and unfairness in relation to doctors' ethnicity and place of qualification (details on the GMC website). I add to this locum doctors as a specific group[23]. (Episode 10, "Better Half", see page 195).

Responses to freedom of information requests revealed that between April 2010 and September 2018, the NHS sacked 10,604 members of staff under the SOSR (Some Other Substantive Reason) mechanism. These were commonly justified by a breakdown in relationships. The current law requires whistleblowers who claim they have lost their jobs due to their disclosures to meet a series of legal tests, which invite the employer to attack whistleblowers, for instance by casting aspersions on whether they genuinely acted in the public interest. "If any [test goes] wrong, your case fails entirely," [25]

The non-medical wife of an anaesthetist, who committed suicide after being referred to the GMC, led the group Voice of Doctor's in a survey in 2022. There were 548 respondents. I have her permission to reproduce the summary slide of the data here:

Questions	% agreed
1 Independent scrutinising body looking at referrals	90.1
1 Referrals should be anonymised (reduce discrimination)	90.1
2 GMC should be held to legally enforceable timelines	98.5
2 There should be an ability to request an accelerated investigation	98.3
2 GMC should not be circulating sensitive info about doctors to their employers prior to investigation	76.6
3 Change standard of proof back to criminal (beyond reasonable doubt)	86.5
4 The GMC should not run an investigation after the police or jury have found the doctor not guilty	72.4
5 There should be an accessible way to appeal unfair interim orders	93.1
6 There should be a method to claim compensation if the doctor has been unfairly treated by the GMC	98
6 There should be scrutiny of the GMC if they have mistreated a doctor	96.7
6 There should be a dedicated tribunal to hear complaints of discrimination	97.5

Thursday, 21st November 2024

HCSA
The hospital doctors' union

The GMC process from referral is very slow and difficult to challenge once commenced. In my experiences, the effect of having a lengthy investigation hanging over means you are often forced to continue working in an environment which may have given rise to the referral in the first place.

The culture in the NHS perpetuates this. The GMC has also unlimited powers as shown by the unwillingness of the courts to overturn decisions. The GMC has oversight by the Professional Standards Authority (PSA), but in reality the PSA has no legally binding role and the GMC appears to act independently. The context in which the doctor is accused is not necessarily reflected in the round when making a referral or when an expert prepares a report. Commonly the doctor is expected to perform unsupported with unworkable job plans, bullying by management, intimidation of witnesses (chaperones, secretaries, colleagues) with threat of disciplinary action if they give statements in support, and no account taken of these factors or mitigating personal circumstances. This is more likely to happen in a locum where the doctor is not known.

On 15 February 2023, Dr Sheena Meredith wrote in *Medscape UK*, about The General Medical Council's (GMC) pledge to act upon recommendations made by its internal review of November 2022, of its processes into how it "monitors for and mitigates against bias in its decision making"[26,27]. Co-chaired by Professor Iqbal Singh CBE and Martin Forde KC, it found that the GMC "incorrectly applied the legal test" in considering the allegations against Dr Arora[28], and that the allegation of dishonesty "should not have been taken forward". The GMC had "missed multiple opportunities to stand back and assess whether the allegations were serious enough to be referred to a tribunal", the review concluded. "The case raised once again the perception of a regulatory process lacking in fairness; of a system in which the stakes seem much higher if you are a black and minority ethnic doctor."

Dr Yasotha Browne, equality, diversity and inclusion lead at DAUK told *Medscape UK*, "What happened to Dr Arora was in the open arena, meaning many people and bodies were participants including the GMC. We think this highlights an illiterate anti-racist culture. Given that 25% of our NHS workforce is foreign born, this is a terrible concern for welfare and rights. Charlie Massey's apology should be followed by seismic change to restore trust, that is what is critical. These concerns were echoed by the British Medical Association (BMA), whose Council Chair Professor Philip Banfield described the report as "damning." He said: "This one case lays bare significant flaws in the GMC's fitness-to-practise processes and decision making."

The doctors' regulating body said the 23 recommendations "are now being taken forward, with some already in progress". (Episode 11 "Capybara", see page 195. Introduces new challenges for the club, including legal troubles.)

The internal review, a 27-page report, follows a long series of controversial decisions by the GMC – many of which were followed by their dedicated internal review. It resulted in extensive criticism of its handling of fitness to practice cases, which led to multiple accusations of and saw the regulator labelled as 'dysfunctional' and 'not fit for purpose'[22,23] (See e-mail 11.11.22 in Medscape ref. GMC)

The internally commissioned review, to which the GMC said over 40 GMC and Medical Practitioners Tribunal Service (MPTS) staff substantively contributed, with an additional 900 'colleagues' that contributed via surveys, focus groups, team meetings, and one-to-one interviews, made recommendations covering five main areas:

1. A more consistent approach to the GMC's auditing of the fairness of its work, including seeking more external feedback
2. Increased consistency across the organisation, with the introduction of a single set of decision-making principles
3. Equality, diversity, and inclusion (EDI) training for GMC staff to be tailored across different roles
4. More detailed data about GMC fitness to practice processes to be published
5. Ensure fairness and EDI are embedded into the way the GMC operates in future when the Department of Health and Social Care introduces a new regulatory framework for healthcare professionals. Top of Form (See Episode 12, "The Sleep of Babies", page 196. Deals with the consequences of the past.)

The relationship between the workforce, whistleblowing and employers, is a subject of great interest in exploring the relationship and the interactions of the law, medical ethics and towards a better understanding of the working within various institution[28,29]

2010 Scotland fraud inquiry and my exoneration

Sharmila Chowdhury: Radiology service manager at Ealing Hospital trust - Sacked after blowing the whistle on senior doctors who were moonlighting at a private hospital while being paid to treat NHS patients. Suspended after a counter-allegation of fraud made against her by a junior whom she had reported for breaching patient safety. The allegation was never proven and in July 2010 the employment tribunal judge took the unusual step of ordering the trust to reinstate Ms Chowdhury's full salary. However, the trust made her post redundant, and the case was eventually settled out of court

I ran single-handed a cardiology unit in the Vale of Leven for four years when part of Argyle and Bute Health Board. In October 2004 I took up the post. I replaced Dr. Al-Khafajy immediately following his move to another post. I worked as a single-handed cardiologist and ran the cardiology service at the Vale of Leven Hospital.

I initially contracted for a three-month locum, but it was repeatedly extended until it ended in December 2007. I commuted every Monday morning on the early flight on EasyJet from Bristol to Glasgow. I negotiated a four-day week returning Thursday night, except every sixth week, when I was the on-call consultant over the weekend. I lived in hospital accommodation and since there were no kitchen facilities, would eat out. Before going out I would get some exercise, half an hour swimming a few lengths in the local pool. Some evenings I would go to watch a film. I had a membership with the Vue Cinema in Glasgow city centre.

This became a long-term locum commitment pending reconfiguration of services in Glasgow Health Board. I was on call for general medicine 1:6 and I was resident in the Vale of Leven during the week. I was involved with a pilot study, the "Lomond Integrated Care Project" evaluating an acute medical service involving GPs when the new FY1 and FY2 juniors replaced the current medical SHOs. I had weekly sessions in the Western Infirmary Catheter Laboratory Glasgow, where I did three or four 'radial' cases and pacemaker implants as required. I had occasional commitments in other Argyll and Clyde hospitals including in pacing lists at The Royal Alexander Hospital in Paisley and angiograms at Inverclyde Hospital in Greenock. I attended the Wednesday morning joint cardiothoracic meetings at the Western Infirmary to discuss cases. I set up a weekly stress echo service on a Vivid 7 system (GE Vingmed) at the Vale of Leven. My yearly appraisals were with Dr McCruden. I inherited a small private referral base and secured admitting privileges at the Nuffield and BMI Ross Hall Hospitals Glasgow. I continued to run my clinics in Glasgow for several years after I left the locum.

It was 2004 and influenced by the entrepreneurial spirit of my father (author of *Entrepreneurship: The Seeds of Success*) while in Glasgow, I started a novel remote monitoring service using the emerging telemedicine technology (the Docobo Hub) to manage patients remotely (https://www.youtube.com/watch?v=0Mi3BTmJ2E8&t=1s). I was diagnosing and treating cardiac conditions (e.g. blood pressure, palpitation, heart failure, angina) and associated co-morbidities (diseases such as diabetes, COPD) in patients while in their homes, or when they were travelling to relatives. I remember one unique patient with cardiac, neurological and gastrointestinal problems who wanted me to look after her when she travelled to Australia for six weeks. She required frequent changes in medication due to the extreme heat there to manage her symptoms and control her blood pressure and arrhythmia and using the Hub I monitored her remotely from the UK. I also gained experience in monitoring my patients following hospital discharge after cardiac surgery and in so doing, shortening the length of their hospital stay. One other memorable case was an elderly patient in Glasgow who did not want further cardiac intervention following a complex angioplasty procedure (stenting of her coronary arteries) for angina with a prolonged hospital stay due to vascular complications (major bruising in her groin - a large painful haematoma) and I offered her my Docobo Hub. From Glasgow, or my home when in Bristol and wherever I was in the UK, I advised her on her blood pressure medication, improved her BP control, in turn her angina, and, importantly, I managed to improve her blood sugars as her diabetes was poorly controlled. Using my telemedicine and my interventions, I prevented further hospital admissions. She was absolutely delighted, as indeed was her daughter who was previously a nurse in the community and was fretting daily about her mother until she was monitored. It was and today remains my frustration that all my attempts to persuade the NHS locally and nationally (I could not even convince the benefits of my cardiology colleagues managing heart failure) to take on this service, fell on deaf ears (See transcript of my Interview with Nick Ferrari on LBC 17.05.24). Trying to get someone interested is hard, even when pilot studies that have shown the benefit, *unless you have got* a champion in the trust and the funding there. Funds appeared for a pilot study, which showed a reduction in admissions of patients with respiratory disease, but there was no one to champion it; the interest went, and funding stopped, ending a valuable service. I think there are several reasons. People have got to be on board with the concept, and a lot of people have their own ideas, and they're not willing to take advice from someone who is outside their little area or their speciality, or outside of their Trust. There may be some funding pressures, obviously for the different things, but it's very difficult to introduce something as an individual unless you have the strong backing of your cohort of colleagues for a pilot study. I presented to my colleagues in the Cardiac Society and GPs, good evidence for using telemedicine to manage heart failure patients out of hospital. You try your best, as an individual it's very difficult and it's interesting how the COVID-19 pandemic has made it blossom because people were forced into having to follow the need and I think the inertia. You're talking about 20 years of potential inertia and even if we said OK, a reason is we haven't had the full evidence for the last ten years, that's still a long lead time, time to get in innovation. (Dr Rasoul from Liverpool University Hospitals presented an almost identical trial to my service at the 2025 British Cardiovascular Society meeting, 20 years after my proposal!). Compare now the situation in 2023 and 2024 following the COVID-19 pandemic.

There is an explosion of this exact service provided via Docobo Ltd, driven by the persistence of Adrian Flowerday, the founder of Docobo and innovative cardiac physiologist, Peter Levene. Since then, growth of the service has been exponentially boosted, initially with the urgent need for patients to isolate from the COVID-19 virus during the pandemic and now sustained by the lack of hospital beds. This under provision of beds has been a longstanding issue due to the loss of around 25% of hospital beds over the last 20 years and simultaneously, the under provision of community support to enable discharge of patients from hospital when 'medically fit' (so-called 'bed blockers') and leading to ambulances stacked up outside emergency departments. On the positive side at least, I have the satisfaction my vision was 20 years ahead of the curve!

The Vale of Leven was absorbed into Greater Glasgow when the boards were merged. I was previously head-hunted to move to a nearby hospital in Paisley however preferred to stay, but when the hospital was taken over by Glasgow Health Board I was unexpectedly accused of timesheet fraud.

This was not the case and my colleagues who signed off my time sheets each week knew this.

However, their assertion I did not submit false timesheets was not accepted by the Health Board, despite evidence Dr McCruden provided to support me. Locums are not suspended on pay (garden leave – a so-called neutral act!) unlike the situation for substantive consultants, when under an investigation, so I was sacked.

My accommodation was in the Vale of Leven Hospital and I was told to leave with immediate effect. That day I rang Dr Paul Mackintyre, my colleague in Glasgow, and the overseer of services as the "Heart Tzar" in Scotland.

I found out what a good friend means in a crisis, as no sooner had I explained my predicament, notwithstanding that Paul and Kate had recently moved house, Paul invited me over and I was given a spare room to stay and filled it with all my hurriedly packed belongings. I recall they had not fully moved in themselves with unopened boxes around, plus his wife had recently been ill and they had young children to look after! Despite my unexpected arrival, I was welcomed into their home and am forever grateful for their kindness. Since then, they moved to Tasmania where Paul expanded cardiac services including new interventional pacing services.

Paul sent this testimony on the next page to my solicitor.

Following my sacking from the Vale of Leven, I lost income and was unemployable for a year, while the board referred me to Fraud Scotland. My medical defence union and GMC were necessarily involved, and I eventually found myself attending a hearing in Manchester where the full facts were presented and I was cleared.

At the time I was not offered a transcript of the proceedings (it would require a stenographer to type one up on request) so on 18 March, 2025, I made an FOI request. However, my hearing was over seven years ago and Fraud Scotland did not reply to my request. The General Medical Council is also unable to provide a transcript as the GMC only retain recordings of hearings (which are used to produce transcripts) for seven years. To fulfil commitments to processing personal data in line with data

CLYDE DIVISION
MEDICAL DIRECTORATE
CONSULTANT: DR PAUL D MACINTYRE

Royal Alexandra Hospital
Corsebar Road
PAISLEY
PA2 9PN

NHS
Greater Glasgow and Clyde
1948–2008
60 years of the NHS

Date: 23.11.09
Dictated 23.11.09
Ref: PMI/AMC

DIRECT ☎:Secretary - 0141-314 7097

TESTIMONY FOR DR LANCE NICHOLAS FORBAT

Dear

I have known Dr Lance Nicholas Forbat for approximately five years. He was appointed as a Locum Consultant Cardiologist to replace Dr Al-Khafajy at the Vale of Leven Hospital in Greater Glasgow and Clyde Health board. I met Dr Forbat at the Western Infirmary where he was performing his weekly coronary angiography list. He also brought patients to the Royal Alexandra Hospital for permanent pacemakers. I did not work with him directly but I believe him to be competent to perform these procedures.

Over the course of the last five years I have had many conversations with Dr Forbat regarding his work at the Vale of Leven Hospital, with regards to patients and his commitment to service development.

He is a highly motivated individual who was well regarded by is consultant colleagues and also his colleagues in cardiac physiology at the Vale of Leven hospital. In my opinion he worked very hard during his consultant post. He is experienced in echocardiography and developed a stress echo service at the Vale of Leven Hospital.

It is my understanding that his work plan was agreed with his fellow consultants. The post then became long term and he elected to perform private practice in Ross Hall hospital and the Nuffield Hospital in Glasgow. This would be considered an unusual step for a consultant in a locum position. However his locum post lasted a total of 3 years.

I have met Dr Lance Forbat socially on several occasions and found him to be very enthusiastic about his work. I have no doubt from what he communicated to me that he stayed many evenings at the Vale of Leven and kept himself available to junior medical staff and staff in the minor injuries unit to support their clinical judgement on cardiology matters.

I am happy to provide a testimony for Dr Lance Nicholas Forbat to the best of by knowledge when he was a locum consultant cardiologist at the Vale of Leven hospital.

Yours sincerely

Paul D MacIntyre

Dr Paul.D.MacIntyre
Consultant Physician & Cardiologist

RECEIVED
26 NOV 2009

16

protection legislation, at this point recordings are permanently deleted. The key paragraphs from the determination by the GMC are reproduced below:

Investigation Committee (Oral hearing)

Dr Lance FORBAT

Reference Number: 2647328

16 December 2009

St James's Building, 79 Oxford Road, Manchester M1 6FQ

The Committee has read the testimonials which were submitted on your behalf by Mr Lazarus. They are all supportive of you and show that you are held in high regard by your peers including consultants at the Vale of Leven Hospital and those you currently work with. One member of Argyle and Clyde Health Board comments that you were very highly valued at a time when the acute services were under threat. He further states that he has found you to be a man of both loyalty and integrity.

The Committee has carefully considered the issue of proportionality when deciding whether it would be appropriate to issue you with a warning. The Committee has in mind the GMC's duty to act in the public interest, which includes the protection of patients and maintenance of public confidence in the profession. Taking all these factors into account the Committee is satisfied that it is neither appropriate nor proportionate to issue you with a warning and directs that no further action be taken.

It is accepted that you could have completed the timesheets with more information. However, the Committee finds that there is no evidence that you were any more than careless. The format of the timesheet was also not conducive to being completed in a satisfactory manner.

The Committee accepts that there is no evidence that you were undertaking any private angiograms as alleged in Paragraph 7 of the Notice of Hearing dated 10 November 2009.The Committee has been given no evidence that you were required to inform the Trust of any private work you were undertaking. The Committee also accepts that you worked in excess of the hours that you claimed for and is satisfied that your actions were not fraudulent or dishonest.

No further action was needed, and I was cleared. I was able to get a locum in Dumfries and Galloway and informed both the agency and new employer of the reasons why I was dismissed from my previous post at the Vale of Leven. On 31 December, 2007, my contract with Dumfries was terminated by the agency in response to a letter from Greater Glasgow Health Board! I, however received support from Ian Miller, the Chaplin of the Vale of Leven and was reinstated:

From: Ian Miller
Date: 31/12/2007 19:58:31
To: lance.forbat@doctors.org.uk

Hi,
I have written to Angus McKay as follows..........

I have spoken to Dr Lance Forbat today. I am only hearing his side of the story but I do know that he is well respected in the hospital and the patients I have spoken to all have a high regard for him. They also feel that his attention was, in their opinion, usually beyond the call of duty. I therefore find it interesting that GGHB allege that he was somehow cheating them. He comes over as a very honest guy. Bottom line is that he seems to have been pronounced guilty without a trial. It occurs to me it is just another way of ruthlessly sounding the death knell for the Vale.

The Health Board have also written to Dumfries and Galloway trying to ensure that they do not continue to employ him. He has kept the service going for the last few years and it suits GGHB to see the back of him. I think it is grossly unfair. I am now probably sounding paranoic!

I visited a friend today in WD 4 and it just brings home to me just how much we value this service. The place was heaving. It will be a bad 2008 for our community if GGHB gets their wishes. I wish you well for the New Year. I am off to Tenerife with wife, son, daughter in law and grandson. You take care and thanks once again for all you have done and all you may yet do and for giving us some hope. Though we appreciate that the Health Board is a very powerful and influential adversary.

It may be not much but I do know Angus and he knows that I know the staff. He will know I speak the truth when I speak of the high regard people have for you locally. He is also well aware as to just how duplicitous the Health Board can be.

I spoke to Graham Tait and found him very open and supportive. I am sure that he will do everything he can. He is quite sure that you have been treated unfairly. If I can do anything further or speak for you in any way please let me know. I hope that 2008 will start better than 2007 ended.

Take Care. Ian Miller

I was delighted to receive this letter from The Members of the Community of the Vale of Leven addressed to me at Dumfries Hospital. I had no contact with them during my locum and indeed was not aware of the group's existence.

Members of the Community
Vale of Leven Hospital

14th Jan 2008

Dr Forbat
Dumfries Hospital

Dear Dr Forbat

We felt we had to write to you after reading the article in the paper
We are so sorry to hear what has happened to you
We note also that Jackie Pollock is condemning the Health Board and appears to be sticking up for you

That is just Jackie You are a lucky person to have her on your side

Some of us who decided to write this letter to you have actually been your patients and we found you a great doctor Kind and understanding to your patients

Since we read the article in the paper we have been talking to some staff at the hospital and to folks who know Jackie

They tell us Jackie is supporting you all the way and they also say you are in contact with her on a regular basis She will do all she can for you
We have had feedback from people who have met Jackie and she is telling all you are not guilty of anything Good on her

We do not know how well you know Jackie but she is just our Jewel in the Crown
From the start of services being removed from the Vale Jackie has campaigned to save them
She took on arranging public meetings to which we all went and this has been since 2003 She has taken on our local MSP and she took on Argyll and Clyde Health Board
Now she is taking on Greater Glasgow
We know one of our local GP's Dr Trust has great admiration for Jackie
At one public meting last year over 1000 people turned up and some still had to be sent away

Can we say to you put you trust in Jackie Not once has she ever got anything wrong as she checks her facts thoroughly
She always jokes that one day she will end up in jail for all she does

WE are all very fond of Jackie and were devastated when she nearly lost her life in 1998 during a Cancer operation in the Vale
That did not keep Jackie down Once recovered she started a Breast Cancer Support Group so people could have support after their ordeal of cancer Jackie also told her story to large meetings of MacMillan Cancer Support

Dr Douglas McCruden was the diabetologist and the lead physician at the Vale, who signed off my timesheets and gave this reference.

NHS Argyll & Clyde

DEPARTMENT OF MEDICINE

Consultants: Dr D C McCruden
Dr H A Carmichael
Dr L N Forbat (Locum)
Dr M R Al-Shamma
Dr F A Johnston

Vale of Leven District General Hospital
Main Street
Alexandria G83 OUA
Tel: (01389) 817241
Fax: (01389) 817319
E-Mail : Davina.Kenny@vol.scot.nhs.uk

NHS
Argyll
& Clyde

DCMcC/DK

23 July 2008

Ms Ewelina Oskroba
ID Medical
Norfolk House East
499 Silbury Boulevard
Central Milton Keynes
MK9 2AH

Dear Ms Oskroba

DR LANCE FORBAT

Lance Forbat worked as Locum Consultant Physician with a special interest in Cardiology in this Department between October 2005 and December 2007. In terms of Cardiology, this is a single handed specialty post. The General Medicine commitment involved one in six acute medical receiving. Dr Forbat had Clinical Lead responsibility for CCU and the rest of the hospital's cardiac service. He carried out one coronary angiography session weekly with less frequent pacemaker implantations. The service he provided was excellent in all respects. He was an extremely good colleague to work with. He was proactive, energetic and prepared to be deeply involved in all aspects of the running of our Unit. I thoroughly recommend him both as a General Physician and a Cardiologist.

His locum here was terminated by management because of what were seen as irregularities in the filling in of his timesheets. I am now happy to have been informed by Dr Forbat that his representatives have been told that no prosecution is to be undertaken.

Yours sincerely

D C McCRUDEN
Consultant Physician

This is a true certified copy of the original. No visible alterations have been made by an unauthorised person.

Date: 2 4 JUL 2008

Signature: ....

Position: COMPLIANCE OFFICER

After the outcome of the investigation by Fraud Scotland, Dr. Hugh Carmichael gastroenterologist at the Vale, sent his letter.

On 3 January, 2008, I was reinstated in the post at Dumfries.

NHS GREATER GLASGOW
& CLYDE
DEPARTMENT OF MEDICINE

Vale of Leven Hospital
Main Street
Alexandria G83 OUA
Tel: (01389) 817239
Fax: (01389) 817319

1948–2008 60 years of the NHS

Consultants:
Dr D C McCruden
Dr M R Al-Shamma
Dr H A Carmichael Enquiries to: Dr Carmichael's Secretary
E-Mail: Angela.Smith5@nhs.net

Dr F Johnston, Department of Medicine for the Elderly

HAC/AS

8TH DECEMBER 2008

TO WHOM IT MAY CONCERN

REFERENCE – DR LANCE FORBAT

Lance Forbat served here as Locum Consultant Physician and Cardiologist from November 2004 until December 2007. During his three years with us we all found him to be a highly experienced, hard-working and committed member of the Acute Medical Team. His general medical and cardiological skills were exemplary. He provided and developed an excellent cariological service both to ourselves and to other departments within the hospital. He made himself available to juniors and seniors for advice and help.

As well as his clinical skills in acute medicine and cardiology he supervised and undertook cardiological assessment including echocardiography, trans-oesophageal echocardiography and, in the Western Infirmary, Glasgow, undertook coronary angiography on appropriate patients on a weekly basis and participated in the clinical meetings with other Cardiologists on that site.

We all found him friendly, approachable and available. He took an active interest in the educational needs of the junior doctors and sought to develop services as appropriate during his time with us.

I have every confidence in his abilities and I am sure will not be found wanting should he be successful in his application.

Yours sincerely

DR H CARMICHAEL
CONSULTANT PHYSICIAN

Chapter 12

2021-23 GMC investigation, the lengthy process, assessment and conclusions

This episode in my career occurred between 2018 and 2019 when my personal circumstances were at an all-time low. My parents were ill at 87 and 89 and we were selling their home to pay for long-term care. My mother had worsening dementia, and my father had several admissions to hospital with heart failure and failed discharges. My brother, only 14 months older than me, had terminal liver cancer and his condition was deteriorating rapidly. Both my father and then my brother died within three months of each other, followed four months later by death of an uncle. During this period, I was travelling two hours daily each way to work and also visiting my parents. I was dealing with the deteriorating physical condition of Dad, as well as with Mum developing early signs of dementia and implications for moving into a care home and then selling their home. For a few weeks I lived in their empty house, sleeping in a sleeping bag on a blow-up bed, pending completion of a sale, to be near my locum in Homerton Hospital and their care home in Weybridge. Each evening after work I would be sorting out the house contents with family helping on weekends. Around this time Dad's care during admissions St Peter's Hospital was suboptimal, leading to readmissions with either fluid overload or the opposite, dehydration leading to renal failure. Sandra and I were doing our best to communicate our concerns with the responsible consultants and ward staff, but we were ignored despite being consultants with considerable experience, including my specialist interest in heart failure. We eventually insisted on an inquiry. Sandra and I were exasperated by the Trust's failure to answer questions, failure to employ an independent investigator to review the issues, and the delays (it took over a year). I was invited to meet the Chief Executive and board members and in my professional experience of such meetings, this was a farce, with denials and an attempt to cover up! I was astonished, as a cardiologist with decades of experience in managing heart failure, to be told by a consultant chest physician, in front of those attending including the CEO (a qualified nurse) and lay members present representing the Trust, that weighing patients (the lack in Dad's case was evident in his repeated re-admission) is not essential or reliable in managing heart failure! Eventually we went to the NHS Ombudsman, and this was delayed by the COVID-19 pandemic too! In the final analysis the Ombudsman upheld most of our complaints listed below, but not all, as they engaged a general physician and his opinion differed from ours. (Dad's final report is not published when I searched at https://decisions.ombudsman.org.uk/ and is reproduced in the appendix). Thus, despite my cardiology experience, this was not enough to override their expert's views in all key areas of contention.

In memory of our Dad, who I promised I would never give up striving for the truth and improvement in care for patients, I share here the outcome of our efforts.

Parliamentary and Health Service Ombudsman 10.06.22

Complaints upheld:

We have identified some failings in the care the Trust provided during the first admission in 2018. This may have contributed to Mr. Forbat's need for a further hospital admission.

We have also identified a failing in the Trust's complaint handling.

Mr. Forbat had heart problems and had been taking diuretics (water tablets). The Trust stopped and restarted them during his admission. When it discharged Mr. Forbat on 18 January, it did not prescribe further diuretics.

Mr. Forbat returned to hospital on 15 February 2018 with chronic heart failure. The Trust discharged him on 8 March and he sadly died on 28 March. Drs Forbat complained to the Trust about the care it had provided. The Trust aimed to respond in May.

When Dr Lance Forbat contacted the Trust in June, it acknowledged there had been a delay in reviewing the complaint. In December 2018, the Trust concluded the reviewer it had appointed had not carried this out.

In March 2019, the Trust met with Dr Forbat and appointed a clinician to carry out the independent review. It shared this with Drs Forbat in June 2019 and later met with them to discuss this.

The Trust acknowledged 'Mr. Forbat's admission on 15 February 2018 with acute exacerbation of chronic heart failure could have been potentially avoided at this stage. A combination of suboptimal discharge planning during admission in January 2018 and a lack of continuous community care led to a delayed start of oral diuretics at suboptimal dose.

National guidance from the GMC says doctors 'must adequately assess the patient's conditions, taking account of their history and promptly provide or arrange suitable advice investigations or treatment where necessary'. In line with this the Trust should have assessed Mr. Forbat, put in place a management plan and arranged treatment.

Section 7.3 of the NICE guidance on chronic heart failure says 'all patients with chronic heart failure require monitoring. This monitoring should include:

- *a clinical assessment of functional capacity, fluid status, cardiac rhythm (minimum of examining the pulse), cognitive status and nutritional status*
- *a review of medication including need for changes and possible side effects*
- *serum urea, electrolytes, creatinine and eGFR*

(Monitoring also specifically includes heart rate control, blood pressure including postural changes (lying and standing or sitting if not standing) with daily weights as essential measurements.)

(On 6th January 2018 father was hypotensive, BP 79/54mmHg and remained so over 24hrs. On 7th recorded as 85/56mmHg. On 8th January .. advised restarting diuretic if renal function improved and on 9th his blood pressure was 100/60mmHg, but no postural blood pressure was recorded. The following day 10th January .....reviewed our father advising for ready his discharge. However on 11th January the records say he was confused. 14th January 2018 he was in a chair and there is reference to 'grade III pressure sores', surely not acceptable just prior to discharge if not managed. He was deemed 'MFFD' on 16th January 2018.

After stopping the diuretics on 6 January, the Trust restarted Mr. Forbat on a smaller dose (40mg furosemide daily) on 14 January. Mr. Forbat received this dose until he was discharged on 18 January. He was also on spironolactone 25mg to be restarted when renal function stable.)

The Trust should have ensured Mr. Forbat was monitored in line with the NICE guidance to make sure the dose he was receiving was clinically effective. Based on the records and the clinical advice we received, there is no evidence this happened from 14 to 18 January. This was a failing.

It is difficult to know what the impact of the lack of monitoring was but the crisis which caused Mr. Forbat's February admission may have been avoided. The Trust appears to have broadly acted in line with our Principles. However, there is no indication it has identified the failing in monitoring Mr. Forbat when his diuretics were restarted.

The Trust has acknowledged Mr. Forbat's admission in February could have been potentially avoided if the discharge planning in January had been better.

The complaints correspondence shows Dr Forbat complained in March 2018 and the Trust aimed to respond in May. When he chased this in June, the Trust acknowledged there had been a delay in reviewing the complaint. The Trust said this was due to human error. This delay is a failing.

It was only in December 2018 that the Trust concluded the reviewer it had appointed had not carried this out. The Trust appears to refer to this as an unavoidable delay but there does not appear to have been any correspondence with Dr Forbat between June 2018 and January 2019. This was not in line with our Principles and is a failing.

The report (6th June 2019) is not structured in the same way so some points are addressed more holistically than others. The Trust agreed the report 'was not as detailed as it could have been' There is a failing in communication during the complaints process. We recognise this contributed to Drs Forbat losing faith in the Trust.

Complaints not upheld:

We have provisionally not seen any failings in the care the Trust provided during Mr. Forbat's later admission. We have not identified any failings in the care the Trust provided to Mr. Forbat in February. This is because it appears the care was in line with the relevant guidance.

Patients or their families may have questions or concerns about the treatment. In these circumstances, the Trust should take their views into account. This is what the Trust did when Dr Forbat expressed concerns that his father was dehydrated.

However, 15th to 27th February: it took several visits of family members raising concerns at each that were 'ignored' and/or not responded to appropriately or professionally (often dismissively or rudely) and over a weekend on call when I was concerned about his deteriorating condition, it required me to phone a manager to get a senior opinion, in the event to contact a registrar, to see my father and subsequently it took a direct call from me to the cardiology consultant. Furthermore when I visited the instructions for blood tests were not carried out as the consultant requested.

The complaints correspondence shows Dr Forbat complained in March 2018 and the Trust aimed to respond in May. When he chased this in June, the Trust acknowledged there had been a delay in reviewing the complaint. The Trust said this was due to human error. This delay is a failing.

The Trust has acknowledged the cardiologist who eventually reviewed Mr. Forbat's care provided sessional cardiology care to patients at the Trust. This clinician had not been involved in Mr. Forbat's care. The Trust said the two clinicians it had previously contacted to carry out the review were entirely independent of the Trust but neither could commit to completing this.

Actions:

The Trust carried out an internal investigation into the lack of discharge medication (diuretics). This recommended discharge medication should be checked against the current drug chart.

In February 2019, the Trust published updated Discharge Guidance for patients with Heart Failure, with information about fluid intake, salt, weight, alcohol and symptoms. It includes information about local and national support groups and contact details for the Trust's Heart Failure Nurse.

The report author suggested the Trust should identify two main wards as hubs for patients with acute heart failure and to appoint an acute heart failure nurse. The Trust had a chronic heart failure nurse already and the intention was that these nurses would work between the two hub wards.

The Trust told us it had asked the Cardiology Consultants to consider this recommendation of a heart failure specialty ward outside of the recognised acute unit. The Trust told us it also planned to carry out a heart failure and cardiac specialist nurse/practitioner resource review to identify any gaps in resource provision and/or education.

In line with our Principles, we recommend the Trust writes to Drs Forbat within six weeks of the date of our final (i.e by 17th October) report to confirm which actions it has completed. It should also explain what action it will take, or has taken, to address its failure to monitor Mr. Forbat at the end of the January admission.

In relation to its complaint handling, the Trust should explain what action it will take, or has taken, to address complaints in an appropriate level of detail. It should include this within in its letter to Ashford and St Peter' Drs Forbat and send a copy to us.

As part of our recommendations, we have asked the Trust to write to you by 17 October (2022).

I sent an e-mail to the Senior Caseworker Parliamentary and Health Service Ombudsman on 19 October 2022 08:58 Subject: [External] Re: PHSO's final report on your complaint (C-2002700)

Neither myself or my sister have received any letters from St Peter's CEO due by 17.10.

Reply Sent: 19 October 2022 11:10

...drafts had been approved by the Associate Director of Quality and were due to go to the Executive team for final sign off. It said 'They may not be sent on Monday 17 October 2022, however they will be sent as soon as possible afterwards.'

On 19 Oct 2022, at 13:17:

Dear Drs Forbat

I have an update which replaces what I said initially. The Trust sent a letter to each of you by recorded mail on Monday 17 October 2022.

We eventually did receive it on 20th October!

Letter from Ashford and St. Peter' Hospital NHS Foundation Trust

"Ashford and St Peter's NHS Foundation Trust accepts the findings of the Parliamentary and Health Service Ombudsman that there is no evidence that from 14 to 18 January the Trust monitored your father to make sure he had an effective dose of diuretic medication.

I would like to reassure you that the Trust has taken action and implemented new procedures in the intervening years to prevent similar situations arising in the future.

The Trust is committed to reducing hospital-associated harms and in 2019/20 created a Harms Free Care Team under the leadership of a Consultant Nurse in Harms Free Care, who was the first in the UK.

The role brings together the hospital-associated harms of falls, venous thromboembolism (VTE), pressure ulcers, catheter-associated urinary tract infections and harm associated with poor nutrition and hydration.

The team links with the community partners to build an understanding around harm in hospital and across our local health system.

One of the Team's key projects is improving hydration, and in 2020/21 they introduced a pilot project on one of our Senior Adult Medical Wards. We recognised that inadequate hydration contributes to the development of hospital-associated harms and this was an overarching improvement aim for the team.

We also recognise that your father's discharge letter should have included instructions about his diuretic medication, and whether or not he should continue on the medication post discharge.

We are confident that this oversight would now be prevented with the introduction in May 2022 of a new, integrated digital medical records system. The system known as Surrey Safe Care, is now embedded across the Trust, and had brought together previously disjointed clinical systems.

I am also sorry for the lack of communication during the c…omplaints process, particularly the absence of any correspondence between June 2018 and January 2019.

The Trust has addressed the issues in the report in relation to the complaints process. Early in 2019, the Trust created a centralized Complaints Team under the leadership of the Head of Patient Experience and involvement, to provide oversight and operational management of the team.

Since 2020, the team has been part of the Trust's Quality and Patient Safety department, which has improved communication between clinical and administration investigation teams.

In 2021, a further review of the Complaints Team led to the appointment of Complaints Team Lead, to strengthen operational oversight and expected standards.

We continue to monitor the effectiveness and performance of the complaints process, and earlier this year appointed two interim Patient Experience Co-ordinators to support the team following a period of staff absence.

I am sincerely sorry for the ongoing distress this has caused you and your sister and hope this letter will help bring a sense of closure and peace of mind for your family.

For and on behalf of the Chief Executive

Yours sincerely

Medical director"

A few months after these family deaths I was assigned some locums that turned out to be a bad experience. The first was potentially long-term with no interventional sessions but ended prematurely, interspersed with a second very short one, while looking for the third potentially long-term one offering interventional sessions, that also ended prematurely. In the first and third of these I raised concerns with the medical directors about the high workload and lack of support, following which came complaints from a few patients. Having previously ignored the concerns I raised at the start of the first job about workload including systemic failures, I was given no opportunity to resolve the individual issues at the time (as would be normal practice) that led to the complaint. I therefore could respond in the usual timely manner to diffuse the issues raised and if required make any necessary changes to avoid any recurrence. I was a locum and the management response once again was to accrue a few cases, present them together and terminate my locum contract early. I found the whole episode very distressing. When I went from the first bad experience to the next locum the situation could not have been different. I explained my recent bad experience and there was clear understanding. The job plan was sensible, and I was given the support expected by the substantive consultants there. It was a relief. Little did I know that my next locum experience would be a repeat performance only worse! I will expand on these experiences as an '*unsupported locum*' later.

I openly discussed these with my Responsible Officer (RO) at my appraisals. The second Trust was then involved in discussions with my RO. The result as it was the second time a similar problem arose in a locum, was my RO decided he was not able to know I was a safe doctor and proceeded to refer me to the GMC. It is important to realise here, as a locum, my RO was allocated through the locum agency so had never met me or worked with me in any hospital as is the usual situation in a substantive post, did not know me other than via our Zoom interviews when discussing my appraisals. I admitted that I had made some errors in proofreading letters before they went out and gave my explanations and in one letter I dictated the wrong drug name and hence incorrect dose, however, this was spotted by the GP and also another colleague and corrected, so no harm to the patient resulted (I expand on this later). My RO forwarded the information to the GMC and I had a notification in December 2019 of preliminary inquiries.

I notified all Trusts when I applied and secured a series of cardiology locums around the UK, as far south as Conquest Hospital St. Leonards-on-Sea, and north again after 18 years since leaving, back to Cumbria to work in the Cumberland Infirmary Carlisle, now merged into a single Trust with West Cumberland Hospital in Whitehaven with excellent references.

DEPARTMENT OF CARDIOLOGY

Conquest Hospital
The Ridge
St. Leonards on-Sea
East Sussex
TN37 7RD

28 June 2020

To Whom It May Concern

Re: ***Dr Lance Forbat*** ***GMC No. 2647328***
Post: ***Locum Consultant Cardiologist, ESHT, Feb–Mar 2020***

Dear Sir/Madam

Dr Forbat was employed as Locum Consultant Cardiologist at East Sussex Healthcare NHS Trust between 17 February 2020 and 27 March 2020. I worked alongside Dr Forbat during his placement and have been asked to provide a reference to cover the period of his employment. I have also had feedback from colleagues within the Medical team who he worked with during his time here.

Dr Forbat is an extremely experienced senior cardiologist with a wealth of general cardiology knowledge. During his time at the Trust, his duties included ward rounds of the cardiology inpatients, including providing valuable support to the inpatient Heart Failure service. He also undertook general Cardiology and Rapid Access clinics. His clinical decision-making on the ward and in clinic was of a high standard and demonstrated awareness of the latest national and international guidelines.

Dr Forbat was a pleasure to work alongside, with a cheerful and engaging manner. Informal feedback from patients was positive and he also took time to include and engage with other members of the healthcare team including nursing, physiology and administrative staff.

In addition to his role on the cardiac wards, he also performed some outreach duties on the Acute Assessment Unit and I received very positive feedback from colleagues based there regarding his helpful advice, clear management plans and good working with other members of staff in the multidisciplinary team.

I would have no hesitation in recommending him for future work as a consultant cardiologist and we would happily re-employ him in future should the need/opportunity arise.

Please do not hesitate to contact me if you require any additional information.
Yours faithfully

Dr Andrew Marshall MA MD FRCP Consultant Cardiologist
East Sussex Healthcare NHS Trust

I was uncertain after a year had past if my GMC inquiries were leading anywhere and had fully informed the Trust of my ongoing concern. It was a most rewarding locum when I revisited my old department in Whitehaven and received a warm welcome from every one of those who remained after I left in 2002. There was a new wing and sadly cordoned-off parts of the original build where my department was pending refurbishment. The pacing service angiography service transferred to Carlisle long ago.

DEPARTMENT OF CARDIOLOGY
Newtown Road
Carlisle
CA2 7HY

NHS
North Cumbria Integrated Care
NHS Foundation Trust

Date: 14/10/2020

TO WHOM IT MAY CONCERN

I am enclosing my personal reference for ***Dr Lance Forbat - GMC 2647328***

Dr Forbat started with us on 10.08.20 and finished his locum on 18.09.20. During this time, I found him to be hard working, enthusiastic, willing to help at short notice and patient focused.

He not only performed OP clinics in cardiology, but also took up the busy "Consultant of the week" (COW) role apart from implanting permanent pacemakers. I noted that he was involved with the busy COW roles more frequently than normal and performed more than a few pacemaker implants.

He is an experienced cardiologist who was able to settle in our busy challenging department quite fast. He was able to grasp issues and embrace challenges around Medical admissions, cardiology referrals and ad hoc cross covers.

He demonstrated well rounded patient centred clinical care to our patients. I did not come across any issues with Dr Forbat during his time here and I have no reservation in recommending him to work at any Cardiology centres.

I am happy to be contacted for any further information. Yours sincerely

Dr Madhusudhan Varma MBBS, PhD, FRCP(London), FRCP(Edin)
Consultant Interventional Cardiologist

It then took a further two years before an expert report was sent to the GMC and based on this I had to attend an Interim Orders Tribunal (IOT). I had representation from my medical defence union, however, despite their efforts to convince the GMC I was not a risk to patients, conditions were still imposed on my practice. They required me to have an Educational Supervisor and follow an agreed personal development plan (I already had one for my appraisals and adapted this) and to only take on work with approval of my RO and agreement with the GMC. I could only take on locum contracts for a minimum eight weeks. I required a Reporting Officer on site. My agency sent my CV forward for 40 job applications and all declined me and it was six months before I was able to get back to work and earn any income. This was only possible due to the good fortune that one hospital that employed me the previous year (only three weeks) needed a locum and they felt confident enough to take me on with a Reporting Officer and Educational Supervisor agreed with my RO and the GMC. I was also removed as a recognised provider by most major private insurance companies, i.e., I was no longer recognised as a preferred consultant. I followed the GMC's instructions to the letter with the full backing and support of my Reporting Officer and Educational Supervisor in readiness for the decision on whether I would be released form restrictions on the strength of their reports or if I needed to undergo a formal assessment. This was part of the original agreement to release me from the IOT restrictions.

In total, it took four years for the GMC process to be completed and to reach a decision, when I finally underwent an "assessment" (similar to my experience with the NCAA in 2002) and the assessors were practicing physicians in different specialities to mine. I cannot praise these two doctors enough for their professionalism and the way they undertook their respective roles and in particular the care they took in ensuring that I was looked after, by making sure I was not anxious by taking every opportunity to check I was OK. Their explicit aim was to make the environment such that I could perform at my best in what were very stressful circumstances. If any doctor puts themself in my situation, imagine your whole future career as a doctor was hanging on your performance that day and their assessment. This was in stark contrast to my experience of the 'virtual' remote interrogation by the IOT panel when the GMC representative made his opening statement; '*this doctor is unsafe and needs complete retraining*'! I presume his judgment was based on the belief that the report by their appointed expert was a true representation of all the facts. Conclusions within the expert report depended on which version of events was to be believed, the patients' or mine. I felt I was at a massive disadvantage because I believe that chaperones who could have provided supporting testimony were fearful for their jobs if they wrote statements to corroborate my recollection of events. The Charter was clearly intent on arranging a meeting of Mr. Mayhem and me. It was clear from the outset that none of my supporting evidence, including testimonials from those who had known me for decades and testimonials and references from the locums since 2019 had little influence on the IOT panel.

I was informed by my assessors at the end of my final interview that their report and recommendations would be at least a month away as the assessors had to draft their individual reports, then consult each other to combine them into a final document. They had to adhere to the strict GMC protocols. The report would then be sent to the GMC to check it complied exactly with the required content and presented in the correct format.

I dared not apply for any locums until I knew the outcome of my assessment, so for another few weeks I had no income, Yes it really was the whole month later, when at last I received the report with my assessment:

> "***The team unanimously agreed that Dr. Forbat's performance has not been deficient, and he is fit to practice generally***".

Can you imagine the relief that it was over – for now at least as I had finished my last locum that lasted 13 months. Anything over a year is most unusual for agency locums as Trusts push for doctors to switch from an agency to an NHS locum contract. I needed to find my next locum that paid enough to cover my outgoings and debts I built up during several previous periods of unemployment. I also desperately wanted to be based at home having been away from home every Monday to Friday and weekends foreshortened due to the travel time driving Sunday nights to the hospital and late trips returning home in Friday traffic.

I think that had my assessment been done early in 2020 (assuming they had all the supportive information they needed at that time) having regard to all the intervening excellent references, the outcome of my assessment would be the same. It is very important to realise I had spent much time reflecting on the issues from the time I was aware of the complaints until December 2019 when the GMC notified me of a possible investigation. By now enough time had passed following the loss of my father, brother and uncle, for the bereavement process of three deaths to have reached a point where I no longer felt any effect on my ability to deal with additional stresses and I was surely going to incur these going forward. Furthermore, as this length of time had passed I regained better control of my emotions, which are known to be blunted by bereavement, such as showing empathy and I also made adjustment to my work patterns, so avoiding the risk of fatigue from the need for excessive daily travel. My parents were now settled in a care home and we had sold their house to pay for long-term care.

In the intervening period with many locum placements, there were no issues with my work, supported by excellent references, two excellent 360-degree feedback reports and positive appraisals. Unfortunately, none of this is accepted by the GMC as 'objective' evidence of competence. The decision is based only on an independent expert report from written submissions and no interviews with the doctor, that is, until in my case the IOT interview. Important issues for consideration here are I was a locum and whilst I admit had made some mistakes, before these arose I had also raised concerns about the jobs. I explained within a few days of starting the locum, the job plan was overcrowded with overlapping duties in a meeting with the medical director, and in one locum. On the direct advice from the Medical Director, wrote my concerns in a letter to him. Most critically here, I had no one locally who knew me and could vouch for me and offer support.

In 33 years as a consultant, especially when in my substantive posts as a lead consultant, I have come across this scenario on many occasions and I believe my interventions at the time have prevented harm to patients (e.g preventing unnecessary pacing) It has occurred with consultant colleagues and trainees alike, where mistakes do occur and knowing the individuals this has been managed as a learning exercise for all involved. The doctor is not suspended or sacked for these mistakes.

Ideally an analysis of why and how and reasons are explored and any extra support or closer supervision was arranged if needed. In the cases when a Locum makes similar errors, there is rarely the support or consideration for the doctor (unless already well known by staff) or the circumstances in the round and the reflex response is to deal with the problem by removing the doctor. This is driven by fear of any culpability on the part of the Trust, so they defer the decision to an outside body to deal with the individual concerned. This must result in the RO being informed, where they have to decide if it meets the criteria to refer to the GMC. Of course there may be a direct referral to the GMC. In either scenario, the decision to refer is based on the information provided by the Trust that unfortunately has to be accepted as a *true factual account* by the RO or GMC. The doctor has no means of knowing or challenging this. Amongst the many legitimate referrals, published accounts are highlighting malicious or deliberately false accusations and vindictive referrals to the GMC. All referrals can lead to lengthy and expensive investigations against doctors but those that are unnecessary pose an additional burden and I expand on this theme later.

Unsupported locums

While I was coping with my increasing family commitments and getting good references from locums, it happened when I took on one locum. I soon found that I was expected to work an unsustainable and overburdened job plan, so I raised concerns with the Medical Director at a meeting and on his request sent him a written summary of my concerns. I had no proper induction and no protected sessions for administration as I was also covering acute wards during these timetabled sessions. Unlike the substantive consultants in this setting, I had no office of my own to use or even share or adequate secretarial support placed in a noisy open plan area. After a few weeks, I was informed that a few out-patients complained following letters sent out 'with typos' and I was not made aware for some time after, hence was not given the opportunity to respond. In an open plan office, in the presence of other staff, medical and secretarial, a manager announced to me that 'I was no longer required' and my job ended there. In a substantive post, we all get an occasional complaint and are supported in resolving it by the PALS team, indeed the Trust has a vested interest in the consultant and realises this is part of medical practice.

I had no problem with my next locum which fully supported me and offered a sensible job plan. I explained there were issues with clinic letters and software and delayed letters going out. There was no concern and I left at the end of the locum period booked with excellent references. If the Trust decide to call on Mr. Mayhem and 'weaponise' these complaints to make a case to remove a doctor, it is easy for them to do this.

In the next locum that followed I found myself in an almost identical situation, but it transpired to be an even worse experience. I had a very brief induction by a cardiac surgeon to the dictation software used by the Trust (set up differently from the others with the same version) and had no one secretary assigned to me for 5 weeks. Individual letters in any clinic were in a pool for typists to transcribe. Letters were typed in a random order on different days, often weeks late and each by different agency staff, with poor knowledge of cardiology terminology and some had a poor grasp of basic English. I had no office for several weeks and was 'hot-desking' around the various computers and in some secretarial areas there was incessant music playing and no privacy.

I raised my concerns with management and colleagues and I eventually had a share of an office with another locum, as he was shortly due to leave. Yet again, I was informed that a few out-patients complained following letters sent out 'with typos' and one said did not like my manner. This was not the view of my chaperone observing me in my clinics. I was subjected to bullying by one manager after a patient's relative complained about the letter to the GP. There was also a typo on a patient's weight I dictated correctly in kg (I reviewed my dictation) sent out with an incorrect inflated number, but later and unknown to me, after posting had been corrected on the records by a secretary, which led to a complaint by a relative! The patient had not complained about our consultation at the time. My nurse chaperone and senior sister present were all aware of the patient since all commented on a heavy smell of tobacco on their clothes and they had to fumigate the room after for the smell of stale cigarettes. The chaperone had no concerns at the time about the consultation, however, when I was made aware of the complaint, I asked for my chaperone to give her account. She was approached by a manager and changed her mind, she said because of what her managers had said. I believe she was afraid of the possibility of disciplinary action and losing her job. The outpatient Sister promised to write in support but later withdrew the offer, again I believe it was for the same reason, a possibility of disciplinary action. Mr. Mayhem was in the background once more. As in the other locum, a complaint was received from an unhappy patient who had waited months for an appointment, with some previously cancelled and was not happy they had not seen the consultant they had seen privately and who said in his letter he would see them when switched to his NHS clinic. I as the locum, of course, did not have all their private records available in the clinic.

All these issues could be resolved with good communication and would have been if I had been the consultant in a substantive post. At no time did anyone ask how I was, if I had any personal issues at the time that might affect my work, interaction with patients, or any other issues that might have relevance. Other than the Medical Director in the first Trust and department manager in the second, who were made aware because of concerns I raised about the overburdened job plan and lack of secretarial support, no one asked about my insights or concerns. Despite my seniority and experience always with excellent references, there was no interest in why I made these mistakes or how, if I thought there were systemic reasons why I might not be performing at my best. I was however, aware it was common knowledge in the close-knit network of my cardiology colleagues, that I had been a long-term locum since being sacked from Weston General and was a 'whistleblower'. In the one Trust, I was concerned, as the CEO had been in post during both the Stafford scandal leading to the Francis Inquiry and Walsgrave Hospital Coventry following whistleblowing by Dr Raj Mattu, resulting in his suspension and decade-long battle for reconciliation and compensation for false accusations, including over 200 malicious referrals to the GMC.[15,29]

Chapter 13

The Endgame – Finding Solutions

Who was Aneurin Bevan?

Aneurin Bevan was born on November 15th, 1897, in Tredegar. His father was a miner and he was exposed to the problems of poverty and disease. He had nine brothers and sisters, only six of which survived. He left school aged just thirteen, to go to work in the local colliery. During his time as a miner he became a socialist and he was heavily involved in the 1926 General Strike, emerging as one of the leaders of the South Wales miners. He was subsequently elected as the Labour Member of Parliament for Ebbw Vale in 1929. Despite suffering from a severe stammer throughout his childhood he became an outstanding, charismatic orator, overcoming his stammer by spending many hours practising his public speaking skills alone.

During World War 2 Britain was run by a coalition government and William Beveridge published his Report on Social Insurance and Allied Services, known as the 'Beveridge Report'. It advocated that all people in work should pay a contribution into a state fund that could be used to provide people with subsistence in the form of sickness, medical, maternity, old age, unemployment, widows, orphans, industrial injury and funeral benefits.

Labour won a landslide victory in the 1945 general election and their manifesto promised a health care revolution influenced by the Beveridge report. Prime Minister Clement Attlee appointed Bevan as the Minister of Health and Housing and gave him the mammoth task of creating a new 'National Health Service'.

The core principals at the time the of proposal were highly controversial; it should be comprehensive, and meet the needs of everyone; that it should be universal – free to all at the point of delivery to access GP consultations or hospital treatment and that it be based on clinical need, not ability to pay.

Bevan faced bureaucracy, inadequate funding and angry opposition from the Conservative Party and the British Medical Association (BMA). There was even division within the Labour Party itself. Bevan became very embittered but was undeterred and eventually won the support of the medical profession by allowing the consultants to both work inside the NHS and treat their lucrative private patients at the same time.

The Birth of the NHS

On July 5th, 1948, the NHS was launched by the Labour government. For the first time ever nurses, doctors, pharmacists, dentists and opticians were brought together as part of a single organisation with free diagnosis and treatment for all. The first patient to be treated by the NHS was 13-year-old Sylvia Diggory, who had a serious liver condition.

Life in Britain without the NHS is almost unthinkable now but less than 70 years ago healthcare was something of a luxury. Affordable health care was out of reach for much of the population. A doctor's visit could cost the equivalent of half a week's wages, so most people relied on good fortune rather than medical advice to see them safely through an illness.

Prior to the formation of the NHS Britain's health care system was disjointed, being provided by a mixture of insurance companies, local councils and cash-strapped charities. Access to hospitals and health care was difficult for those from working-class backgrounds. Many people had no formal health cover and self-medicated (as with dentistry this decade!) Any significant illness that required a doctor could cause major financial difficulties for families. In the early 1940s and the austerity of the post-World War II years even more so.

The culture

Roger Davidson: Head of media and public affairs for the Care Quality Commission sacked just before the 2010 general election. The regulator was apparently intent on suppressing negative publicity about the NHS, amid political pressure from then Labour ministers. He became head of media at NHS England.

Today we have lost so much of the vision of the NHS when compared to what I expected to be part of when I entered medical school. There have been many advances and good innovations that have transformed the NHS which we are and should be proud of. However, since its inception the devaluation of and erosion of the professional status of doctors, in part due to years of political interference and restructuring on political rather than evidence-based decision-making, added to this the pressure from the increasing demands from changes in the population number and demographics, financial mismanagement and sheer size of the organization, has led to the working environment becoming a toxic one for many of us. (Episode 13, "The Revelator", see page 196).

I have experienced the inward-looking establishment of the NHS where it has lost sight of its primary function to serve patients and allowed political interference and poor management to proliferate and gradually erode the value of the professionals providing the service. Restructuring and misguided reforms by various governments have led to the loss of '*the firm*' and continuity of care that was the glue and offered a sense of community and pastoral care.

The working time directive has led to disjointed and fragmented teams with inadequate safeguards and quality control that was present when the firm was the basic model and in my experience, the resultant prerequisite for high-quality handovers between shifts does not meet these standards. Furthermore, the move to '*ward-based*' care with patients moved regularly between wards or bays within wards, where juniors are allocated individual bays and often on different days, means patients are under the care of different staff. The inevitable consequence is duplication of effort, increasing chances of errors and reduction in the overall efficiency of the system. The reluctance of juniors to make exception reports (likely worried about references) for overrunning their shifts makes a mockery of the working time directive and hides the real issue of inadequate staffing of the service. Competition for scarce financial resources has led to inappropriate and ill-thought-out decisions by those without the clinical knowledge to make them, or willing to ignore clinician input, which is often driven by political expediency.

Silos have always been an issue between departments and specialities that become entrenched in many hospitals, as exemplified by maternity care as a result of cultural and professional boundaries occurring between doctors and midwives, surgeons and physicians and in well-published cases in some regional cardiothoracic centres, between cardiologists e.g. Aberdeen, and St. Georges[30-35] In 2017, the St Georges Trust received its first NICOR alert showing that there was increased mortality of those patients receiving cardiac surgery at the Trust. An 'alert' is when mortality falls below a line 2 standard deviations below the mean for the peer referenced group of 31 cardiac surgery units in the UK. The Trust was also aware of the deteriorating relationship between cardiac surgeons within the unit, issues of unprofessional behaviour by senior staff and a view both internally and externally that the surgeons were working in 'camps' and dysfunctionally (report, paras 1.4, 6.3 and 8.4.1 mention 'camps' and paras 6.6 and 8.4.1 mention 'toxicity' units) leading to poor outcomes. There is evidence that civility saves lives and a culture change is required to achieve this. So that change can occur there must be ownership of the decision-making at local level based on good practices demonstrated elsewhere. Regular review of practices with full engagement of enlightened management and staff is a prerequisite along with sufficient funding and staffing. Openness and positive attitudes to raising concerns with no recriminations are the solution to so many of the scandals over the decades. Following the recommendations of the Francis Report after the Stafford Enquiry none of the critical changes were made and that has led to similar outcomes of poor care as a regular occurrence[36].

The interventions by politicians when passing legislation, or not doing so and NHS England's attempts to resolve these problems have been lacking. A key example is the inadequate PIDA legislation that is accepted as fundamentally flawed and more recently introduction of the government's Freedom To Speak Up project to which I contributed as a witness and in the process met with Sir Robert to discuss my experiences. It puts Freedom To Speak Up guardians who are subordinate employees in the impossible position of holding their bosses to account, when in reality this means that they must either risk victimisation for doing so, or they do what they are told, against the public interest[36-38]. *(See - "Revelator" cont. on page 186).*In advance of our meeting I wrote listing my points for discussion, following which notes of our meeting were sent to me and reproduced below:

Sir Robert Francis QC
Skipton House
80 London Road
London
SE1 6LH

07.10.14

Dear Sir Francis,

Freedom to Speak up Review. Thoughts from a whistleblower

Thank you for giving me the opportunity to meet and discuss my experiences working in the NHS. I qualified in from St. Thomas' 1980 and in my 9th year as a consultant, I was sacked a week before a year into my second consultant post and 5 months after my suspension for raising concerns. I was and remain a 'whistleblower.' This has affected me and my family ever since and despite this I have felt it my duty to speak out on at least two further occasions, that has in turn resulted in me losing employment

I have made several observations that I believe are the root cause of problems. Following my experience (24 years) I have several suggestions to discuss with you and for you to consider in your advice to the government.

Observations

a. *The NHS has an established culture of institutionalised bullying*
b. *The organization is still driven by waiting lists not clinical outcomes*
c. *Politicians have marginalised consultants over decades, so removing their influence.*
d. *Management posts attract those who are generally;*
    i. *Politically motivated*
    ii. *Bullies*
    iii. *Seeking financial gain - bonuses, enhancing pensions etc*
    iv. *Compliant to the organisation, rather than patient centred*

e. *Trusts managers have systems in place that;*
   i. *Distance them from the clinical impact of decisions*
   ii. *Enable control of information and cover-up*
   iii. *Allow disciplinary actions that suppress openness by;*
      a. *exclusion, often on spurious clinical safety grounds*
      b. *use of overt threats of GMC referral*
      c. *insinuating paranoia or mental illness*
      d. *exclusion for consideration of awards*

f. *Chief Executives, board members are not held to account financially. Trusts were 'above the law ' and still currently appear to be so*

Suggested solutions - my order of importance

a. *Whistleblowers if vindicated**, *should be fully compensated by;*
   i. *Financial compensation reflecting lifelong financial loss and security*
   ii. *Substantial damages for defamation*
   iii. *Published apologies with retractions*
   iv. *Reinstatement in post if desired or an alternative in area of choice*

b. *The CEO and others complicit in any cover-up, fired and to lose their pensions*

c. *Organisation should remove bullies from positions of influence*

d. *Incident reporting systems should be transparent – they are currently not*

e. *Medical training to identify bullying, good leadership, genuine whistleblowing*
   i. *bullying is exclusion as well as harassing vs. good leadership*
   ii. *exclusion of whistleblowers by 'getting in first' on spurious safety grounds*

f. *Medical school selection to include assessing traits of bullying vs. leadership*

*** *The onus should be on the employer to 'disprove' a causal link between whistleblowing and 'a pattern of actions' taken leading up to dismissal.***

i.e. bullying, exclusion and disciplinary actions listed above are a recognised pattern. It is easy for the Trust to exclude a doctor then trawl records to discredit a doctor, refer them to the GMC and argue their case for exclusion.

It should be enshrined in law, that 'a pattern of actions' over time to discredit the whistleblower, before and after exclusion, i.e. used to counter any claim by the whistleblower, is enough evidence to prove detriment.

I have come to these conclusions and made my suggestions as a result of years of personal experiences. Implementing some changes will take time, but immediate redress for past and present whistleblowers by starting with a. and b. above would send the strongest message that the culture must change.

Yours sincerely,

Lance Forbat

Freedom to Speak Up Review

Note of a meeting between Sir Robert Francis QC and Dr Lance Forbat

Skipton House - 7*h October 2014, 930am

In attendance:

Sir Robert Francis QC (RF), Chair of Freedom to Speak Up Review
Dr Lance Forbat (LF), Whistleblower
Joanna Donaldson, Director of Freedom to Speak Up Review
Martin Norman, Freedom to Speak Up Review (note)

Minutes:

1. *LF began by noting that he is currently receiving advice from the Medical Protection Society and that they had advised against discussing any of the details of his case with the review.*
2. *RF assured LF that anything discussed during the meeting would be treated in confidence. RF then outlined the structure of the review before asking LF to set out what details he felt able to.*
3. *LF proceeded to outline his experiences of raising concerns and his suggestions on how to improve the process in the future based on his experiences. Key points included:*
   a. *There is a culture of bullying in the NHS. Sometimes there is jealously/ victimisation about private practice.*
   b. *One of the problems is the managers. Managers are often chosen because they toe the line. They follow whatever the political drivers are and ignore the concerns of staff.*

Younger or inexperienced managers don't often know how to handle senior colleagues.

c. *Most places that need a locum usually have problems; otherwise there would be a permanent doctor in post.*
d. *When starting a locum post there should be a proper induction and introduction from someone trusted by medical, nursing and technical staff. When starting as a locum it's usually in a dysfunctional setting with lots of issues. As a locum you don't know the history and therefore if you do things a bit differently it can lead to misunderstandings.*

   Introductions from a person vested with authority and a proper induction, providing the locum with legitimate authority, i.e. equal if a consultant, could mitigate this.
e. *It is very easy for people to undermine you as a locum because you're not permanent and are unlikely to have previous experience in the trust or be aware of the problems.*
f. *The GMC investigation process is outside of reality sometimes. It can ignore standard practice in the hospital, investigating just one doctor against its standards instead of the whole unit who may have similar practices as the doctor being investigated.*
g. *When raising concerns those involved should first sit down as a group and discuss the situation. This should be in a neutral location. Additionally, it would help to have an external person to go to (with no ties to hospital), who could come to the meeting. This should be a quick process especially in terms of assessing the context of the situation (i.e. bullying) and whether any concerns raised are justified. In the case of a locum it is vital this occurs within 24hrs to avoid hasty and unnecessary termination of a contract.*
h. *If there are no sanctions that make people think about their actions they will just carry on doing it. People can't just light a firework and walk away (e.g. managers moving if whistleblowers are vindicated, they should be fully compensated and anyone complicit in cover up should be removed from post and in future not have similar responsibilities.*

   There should also be retrospective remuneration for those currently suffering loss as a result of whistleblowing and action against those responsible for cover-up at the time. In this way there will be no doubt about who is in the wrong.

J. The system needs to be seen to be fair, but guaranteed protection for whistleblowers.

M N

Accountability

Rebecca Prideaux, Former inspector at Britain's health and care watchdog staff at the Care Quality Commission (CQC) were given inadequate training and that workers were discouraged from taking action when they uncovered risks to the most vulnerable. Mrs Prideaux resigned from CQC in May 2013.

Whistleblowing is a necessary but invariably dangerous action by anyone brave enough to go down this avenue as more often than resolving the underlying issues, results in unfair or wrongful dismissal and all the harm associated with this. [6,15,20,28,32] In May 2013, Public Concern at Work (renamed 'Protect') published a research project 'The Inside Story for Whistleblowers' as told by 1,000 callers, to Public Concern at Work's (PCAW) confidential advice line[5]. From nurses and doctors, teachers and carers, office and factory workers, lawyers and accountants, callers come from all walks of life. From their sample, 29% of callers came from Health (15%) or Care (14%) industries. The common responses from management that whistleblowers experienced were categorised as **i). Informal**: closer monitoring, ostracised, verbal harassment, **ii). Blocking resources**: blocking access to emails, information, training, hours, **iii) Formal**: relocation, demotion, job reassigned, suspended, disciplined, **iv) Dismissa**l, **v). Support**: taking the issue seriously is also categorized as support. 60% of those who called the advice line did not report a response from management (either positive or negative) and the remaining 40% (399 people) mentioned responses from management after raising a concern. Of these 74 (19%) feared or expected a response, 29 (7%) had been threatened by management and 296 (74%) had experienced a response from management. Whistleblowers who raise a patient safety concern were more likely to suffer formal reprisal throughout the journey and less likely to encounter informal reprisal than those raising other types of wrongdoing. More worrying was the observation that those raising a patient safety concern tended to be dismissed at their first attempt to raise the concern. New employees may well be more likely to speak up because they are less likely to accept poor or illegal practices. Fear of reprisal or inertia on management's part or lack of feedback may lead an employee to blow the whistle externally. Whistleblowers often fear losing their job if they raise a concern externally explaining a reluctance to go externally. It is particularly challenging for those who are working with patients, vulnerable adults or children, as they may fear passing on confidential information in breach of their professional duties[4].

Employment tribunals (ET) are not the vehicle to resolve these employment issues and they do not keep contemporaneous records of the proceedings!

From the perspective of Trusts (Charters) when engaged with an ET, the trusts are "arming" with ritual advice from bodies, such as the National Clinical Assessment Service (NCAS), which allows NHS employers to behave abusively whilst claiming that they have sought independent advice. Furthermore threatening or making inappropriate referrals to the GMC as a threat to silence whistleblowers is commonplace (*Letter, Carrie MacEwen Chair GMC 24.05.24 referrals to intimidate.)* The truth is that trust managers can obtain whatever advice they want by tailoring the information they feed to NCAS, the GMC and they can also control the subsequent flow of information back through their organisations. The Freedom to Speak Up Guardian, needs to be independent of the Trust and preferably off-site, essential to maintain confidentiality as it is easy to log who is entering their office especially if on more than one occasion.

Stephen Bolsin was asked what lessons could be learned. "No institution, particularly in healthcare, can ever afford to lose sight of its patients." That was in 1998. So instead of denial, gagging and handwringing following the Francis Report into the Mid Staffs scandal, he proposed how NHS managers and clinicians should respond to the complaints about quality of care.

The cost of doing nothing effective is £2bn each year – the cost to the NHS caused by healthcare errors. I have estimated this could more than double if whistleblowers are fully compensated for their financial losses, the effects on their careers and the long-term harm to them and their families[15,36-38].

Stephen Bolsin proposed four relatively simple, inexpensive measures.

1. An organisational commitment to quality and safety.
Monthly "safety walkarounds" should be conducted at the most troubled organisations.

A series of repeated questions should be asked of care providers.

Examples include: what is the next clinical error likely to be in your workplace?

What barriers to providing good care do you experience most commonly?

What can I do to help prevent the next breach of safety or quality in your work area? What would you do differently if you were caring for a close relative?

The safety walk-around should be followed up by the same executives until the answers indicate that the problems are being solved. After three months, the organisation will be safer.

2. A sincere response to all incident reports.
Most NHS organisations have relatively sophisticated incident reporting systems, which should give warning of systemic problems in delivering safe, high-quality care.

These reports must be acknowledged.

This validates the person who has reported the incident and ensures that potential "near misses" and actual incidents will continue to be reported.

3. Permanent "forcing functions" to reduce error - *put in place pre-conditions or "forcing functions" that will effectively prevent recurrence.*

4. Encouragement is better than criticism
Although not unequivocal proof of the beneficial effect of reward for error-free shifts, the example is indicative of what could be. The chief executive endorses the changes and comments on the outcomes at the safety walkarounds.

Implementing any of these responses would improve patient care and staff morale in the NHS at a time when both are critically needed. It would also demonstrate that the NHS is prepared to care properly and will never again lose sight of its patients.

The most important to change is the PIDA law, there must be the establishment of the newly proposed 'Office of the Whistleblower' and associated new laws making certain all parties are accountable for their actions. The proper professional status of NHS managers needs complete thinking with a regulatory body akin to the Councils of GMC for doctors and NMC for nurses and midwives.

Filling in Datix reports for incidents does not lead to a robust outcome as each submission open to interpretation by parties that may be influenced by other motives of management to protect the institution or favoured individuals within.

Education and the Royal Colleges

Medical education should include in the undergraduate curriculum the importance of Duty of Candour in providing safe medical practice, as exemplified by the example of Stephen Bolsin[39]. It should cover why we need whistleblowers[40-43], explain their role and why they are often perceived as a threat[44-49]. The ethics surrounding the duty of candour could be included[50-53] and an update knowledge of guidelines[54] and the recent mandate from the GMC[54], leading hopefully to the necessary changes in the current law by replacement of the inadequate PIDA law withe new ones with establishment of the independent 'Office of the Whistleblower. The comparison with the aircraft industry and how it has transformed safety is a good comparison to make. Yet when applying it in the NHS, rather than seen as a positive action for reflection, raising concerns often results in unintended negative impact on the doctor (or other healthcare worker) as a result of defensive reactions and retaliation. This comes about by those misinterpreting the concern as either a direct criticism of them or threat to their reputation, the department or the institution. It has had a destructive effect leading to the individual, if pursuing a concern becoming a 'whistleblower' and all the consequences that follow. Students should be expected to know about the recent series of health scandals and the Inquiries and debate these[40,41]. There should be teaching of how these arose, what '*lessons were learned*' and why despite these findings, they are repeated year on year throughout the NHS. I hope the new law will eventually catch up with the reality that Employment Tribunals and the PIDA law are not fit for purpose and the Office of the Whistleblower and new laws will protect the individual before any harm is done to them. There should be accountability at all levels so that no one is under the illusion they can get away with suppressing the truth, bullying, or using all the underhand tactics explicitly designed to undermine anyone who may challenge the system. This is when patient harm is the likely outcome.

The Royal Colleges and Allied professional bodies have a lot to consider. In their roles so far, I find no evidence they have engaged with the problem of whistleblowing (*in contrast to the recent but belated proactive stance by the Royal Colleges on bullying and sexual harassment*) as from my reading it is not in their 'remit' and preferring to defer to the legal profession, or the GMC. But neither of these are without their problems and in my view, they are not the appropriate forum for resolving issues around protected disclosures and the consequences they can have for those that make them. It is not easy for the GMC to efficiently distinguish between the malicious referrals and the genuine referral of a doctor deemed unsafe, or not compliant with good medical practice (GMP). This can be served up by employers in so many different areas covered by GMP that it is a minefield to unpick, especially by the Employment Tribunal. [There has been evidence of lawyers applying inappropriate and adversarial, often (not often but when done is often/ even dishonest tactics) discrimination tactics in cases.] The law in my view currently is not able to protect the whistleblower from these onslaughts.

All managers must have formal training before being qualified to take on the responsibility of running the NHS at all levels and, like doctors and nurses be accountable to a professional body. The government must be clear that changes proposed in reports such as the Francis Report and subsequent enquiries are not buried and forgotten but followed up proactively with sanctions if not carried out. The CQC has not yet shown the ability to proactively uncover problems at an early stage. Sometimes these problems were longstanding, but they did not surface until often many years and several inspections later.

Scenes from a Parallel Universe *Sons of Anarchy*

These scripts were generated in response to scenarios I put into Chat GTP 4

Chapter 4: An Education and More 1974
Episode 1 "Pilot": Introduces the Sons of Anarchy Motorcycle Club, their criminal activities, and the power struggles within the club. Themes include brotherhood and criminal enterprise

<u>Follow on from page 54</u>

Clay: *(Addressing the club members) "Alright, listen up, everyone. We got a business opportunity with the Mayans. It's good money, and it'll strengthen our position in the gun trade."*

Jax: *(Interrupting) "Clay, I've been thinking about this. We've had too much bloodshed lately. The Mayans, the Niners, it never ends. Maybe it's time we consider a different approach. We should focus on our legitimate businesses and make Charming a better place."*

Clay: *(Growing angrier) "Your old man made choices, and they led him to an early grave. You don't want that for Abel, do you? This is who we are, Jax. Don't forget it."*

Jax: *(Resolute) "I won't forget who we are, Clay. But I won't let the club destroy everything we hold dear either. I'll do what it takes to protect my family, even if it means challenging you."*

Chapter 5: Early Impressions 1978

Follow on from page 50

Scene: *A "tense meeting" between Lee Toric and Chibs Telford in a dimly lit bar.*

Lee Toric: *(Entering the bar and approaching Chibs) "Telford, isn't it?"*

Chibs: *(Turning to face Toric, wary) "Aye, that's right. What do you want?"*

Lee Toric: *(Smirking) "I've heard quite a bit about you and your charming little motorcycle club. I'm a collector of information, you could say."*

Chibs: *(Cautious) "Is that so? You should know we don't take kindly to folks poking around where they don't belong."*

Lee Toric: *(Ignoring the warning) "I'm not looking for trouble, Telford. I'm looking for justice. I had a sister. She met an unfortunate end, thanks to your club. I'm here to make sure you all pay for what you've done."*

Chapter 6: Leaders and Losers 1993

Follow on from page 50

Scene: *"The clubhouse", continuing during a club meeting.*

Clay: *(Visibly frustrated) "Jax, we are who we are. We're outlaws, and we thrive on the edge. We can't just go legit overnight. This club was built on the gun trade, and that's what keeps us strong. It's what your old man wanted."*

Jax: *(Defiant) "I get it, Clay. But I'm thinking about our future, about my son. I don't want him growing up in a world of violence and crime. We need to change, make this club something better."*

Follow on from page 64

Episode 2 "Seeds": Focuses on the club's illegal arms trade and begins to delve into the tensions between the club members and their relationships. The episode highlights the strong sense of loyalty that club members have towards one another. The SAMCRO is not just a motorcycle club; it's a brotherhood where members are expected to stand by each other no matter what.

Follow on from page 65

The leader of SAMCRO conspiracy; Clay Morrow, along with his wife Gemma Teller conspired to murder Jack Teller's father, John Teller, because he wanted the Charter he set up with Piney Winston to get out of gunrunning and to run a legitimate business. When the charter arranged for someone to be killed, they voted at the Reaper Table for the person to 'meet Mr Mayhem', a euphemism for putting a contract out to end that individual's life.

SAMCRO Charter was benefiting from the proceeds of gunrunning and become used to controlling the town of Charming by fear and favour and John Teller was about to upset this cosy arrangement. John Teller wrote a diary, and this became a monograph of his thoughts and beliefs in trying to turn around the SAMCRO Charter from crime and violence to make it a better world for his children. One son had already died by this time. The secret of how John Teller met Mr Mayhem was kept from everyone in the Charter, even Piney. Anyone threatening to expose this had their days numbered. The town's Chief of Police Wayne Unser had been groomed by the Charter over the years with backhanders and turned a blind eye to their crimes, however he was desperate to retire and hand over to his deputy, David Hale.

The motorbike gang members are immediately recognisable by their leather biker jackets with the Charter's Reaper logo embossed on them, along with sentiments reflecting their modus operandi and emblazoned with the words 'Mr Mayhem' and 'Sons of Anarchy'. When stripped down bare, they retained their identity in the form of a rather grotesque tattoo of the Reaper covering the whole of their back. Other tattoos were on their arms and torsos. Anyone leaving the Charter had to have these tattoos either written over or surgically removed. Ex-members caught and found not to have done this suffered the consequences of tattoo removal by cutting it out with a knife or burning it off. The Reaper was also carved into a large table that was the focus of meetings (akin to the Trust Board room) where the Charter assembled and voted on any actions to follow and like an auction the decision was finalised by the sound of a wooden gavel on the table.

The leaders of the SAMCRO Charter were Clay Morrow as chairman with Jax Teller as the vice chairman (VC). Jax however had inherited his father's personality and was having an internal battle trying to find a way to turn the SAMCRO into a legal enterprise. SAMCRO was all that he had known since a child, it was as much family as his mother Gemma and stepfather Clay. He was sat next to Clay at the table who, with a rugged appearance of a 'granite' chin and stubble face, held the gavel and Bobby Manson, a stocky bearded man with a large belly sat at the other side at the head end of the table. Around this table, all members were utterly loyal with their own rather despicable characteristics. Tig Trager was 'Sergeant-at-Arms' and he had a streak of violence that even hardened bikers would find difficult to stomach. Chibs Telford had a Glasgow smile from being 'glassed' in a bar and was very loyal to Clay, second only in degrees of violence and deprivation to Lee Toric who ranked below Tig. The roles of the other members of SAMCRO were revealed as the episodes unfolded. Piney Winston required a constant supply of oxygen as he had end-stage emphysema. He was relatively benign and wary of some of the more unsavoury decisions of the Charter and very protective of Jax Teller on the count of his close friendship with his late father.

Rival Charters were always challenging each other for territory in the hope of increasing there their income, however loyalties were flexible when it benefited one side or the other. Who are the losers in this life? In truth everyone lost out, the bikers, the lawmakers, the businessmen and the local people.

If Jax Teller were in charge, the gun-running business could be at risk and, like his father, his position of authority at the table would be weakened. The secrets Clay and Gemma kept from Jax and the others ensured loyalty remained with them. Clay relied on Bobby Manson to look at the larger picture within the charter and watch his back for any dissent, however he needed the likes of Tig and Chibs at the table and Wayne in the community to control his patch effectively. Gemma was outside the charter as the "Old Lady" to Clay, but her scheming and the lengths she would go to protect the club (and Clay) had a major influence on the direction the charter went.

Piney Winston and Jacob Hale Jr, who represent different perspectives and interests:

Follow on from page 65

Jacob Hale Jr: *(Addressing the crowd) "Ladies and gentlemen, we've got to think about the future of our town. We need progress, we need development. The days of relying on outdated industries are over. It's time for a change."*

Piney: *(From the audience, shouting) "Change? You mean selling out our town to big corporations? What about the people who've lived here for generations, like my family? You think we want to see our town turned into a corporate playground?"*

Chapter 7 Snakes and Ladders 1995

Follow on from page 78

The patching-in ceremony ritual involves the sewing of the Sons of Anarchy patch onto their vests, signifying their full membership which reinforces the theme of brotherhood and belonging.

Follow on from page 79

Episode 4 "Patch Over", see page 193, explores themes of loyalty, identity, and the challenges of maintaining the club's code in the face of outside pressure. SAMCRO's decision to patch over the Devil's Tribe is met with resistance from some members who are wary of outsiders joining their ranks.

Chapter 8 Out on a Limb 2002

Follow on from page 102

Episode 5 "Giving Back"

David Hale: *(Entering Unser's office) "Unser, we've got a serious problem in this town, and I don't think you're doing enough about it."*

Wayne Unser: *(Defensive) "Hale, I've been running this police department for years. I know the ins and outs of Charming. SAMCRO is a part of this town, and we've managed to keep the peace."*

David Hale: *(Sceptical) "Keep the peace? Unser, I've seen their rap sheets. These guys are involved in gunrunning, extortion, you name it. They're criminals, and they're running amok here."*

Chapter 9 The Merry-go-Round 2002-2021

Follow on from page 118

Episode 6 "AK-51" delves into the club's arms trade again, highlighting the risks and rewards of illegal activities. Club members are forced to make decisions that go against their personal values, so raising questions about their commitment to the club and the ethical implications of their actions

Follow on from page 123

Episode 7 "Old Bones" reveals secrets from the past and explores themes of trust, betrayal, and the consequences of past actions. The ATF's investigation into SAMCRO's activities remains a looming threat. The authorities are determined to uncover the truth behind the buried bones, and their persistence adds to the overall sense of danger and unease. As the investigation unfolds, it becomes clear that there are secrets and hidden truths within the club that could have far-reaching consequences

Follow on from page 126

Episode 8 "The Pull" explores tensions between the club and other criminal entities, with a focus on the consequences of their actions. ATF's investigation into SAMCRO's activities continues to be a looming threat. The authorities are determined to bring the club down, and their efforts are a constant source of tension and danger.

Follow on from page 127

Episode 9 "Hell Followed" highlights the escalating violence and danger faced by the club members as they become embroiled in conflicts with rival gangs.

"Hell Followed" opens with a violent confrontation between SAMCRO and the Mayans, a rival motorcycle gang. This episode emphasises the ongoing conflicts between the different gangs in the region and highlights the brutal nature of their confrontations. It continues to delve into the internal conflict within SAMCRO, primarily between Clay and Jax. The power struggle between the club's president and the younger, more idealistic member intensifies as they clash over the club's direction and activities. Family dynamics remain central to the storyline. Gemma's loyalty to her family and the club is tested as she becomes increasingly entangled in the power struggle between Clay and Jax. Her actions and decisions have far-reaching consequences for the club and her loved ones.

In summary, "Hell Followed" is an episode that ramps up the tension and violence within SAMCRO and the broader criminal underworld. It explores themes of revenge, loyalty, and the consequences of living a life on the fringes of the law.

Chapter 11 The GMC challenge 2010, 2021-23

Follow on from page 144

Episode 10 "Better Half" focuses on the personal lives of the club members, including their romantic relationships and family dynamics with further character development for various club members, particularly Jax, who faces increasing pressure to bring about change within SAMCRO. It depicts the broader impact of SAMCRO's actions on the local community.

Follow on from page 146

In episode 11 of *Sons of Anarchy*, season one, entitled "Capybara", the series continues to explore the complex world of SAMCRO (Sons of Anarchy Motorcycle Club, Redwood Original) and its members while delving into themes of loyalty, betrayal, and the consequences of their criminal activities. The episode explores SAMCRO's involvement in various illegal activities, including gunrunning and extortion. These criminal enterprises are a major source of income for the club and are depicted as both lucrative and fraught with danger, underscoring the risks they take to maintain their power and financial stability. "Capybara" introduces elements of betrayal and secrets within SAMCRO. As tensions within the club rise, certain members become more willing to act against their comrades' interests, potentially endangering the club's unity and safety. The episode continues to delve into the personal struggles of various club members. Opie's difficulties in reconciling his role in the club with his family life remain a central theme. His strained relationship with his wife, Donna, and the sacrifices he makes for the club are explored in greater detail.

Follow on from page 147

In Episode 12, entitled "The Sleep of Babies" escalates the tension, internal conflicts, and external threats to SAMCRO. The episode continues to explore the internal turmoil within SAMCRO, especially the growing power struggle between Clay Morrow and Jax Teller. Their conflicting visions for the club's future and the leadership of the organisation are central to the episode's plot.

Family dynamics remain a core theme. Gemma Teller-Morrow's role as the matriarch of the club and her intricate relationships with Clay and Jax are front and centre. The tension between her maternal instincts and her loyalty to the club is a central conflict.

It delves into SAMCRO's illegal activities, including gunrunning and extortion, which continue to be major sources of income for the club. These criminal enterprises underscore the dangerous and violent nature of their world. It presents moral dilemmas for club members, particularly Jax, who grapples with the ethics of the club's actions and his own role within it. The consequences of their criminal activities become increasingly apparent, challenging their sense of morality.

Chapter 13 The Endgame – Finding Solutions

Follow on from page 178

Episode 13 "The Revelator" wraps up the first season with intense conflicts within the club and sets the stage for future storylines and continues to present moral dilemmas for club members, particularly Jax. The ethical implications of the club's actions and his role within it are prominent, and the consequences of their criminal activities become inescapable.

It brings to light crucial revelations and secrets that have been simmering throughout the season. These revelations have far-reaching consequences for the club and its members, leading to intense confrontations and resolutions to ongoing conflicts, both within the club and with external threats on the future of SAMCRO and its members.

Articles and Reports and Public Inquiries

Newspaper articles on Weston General Hospital

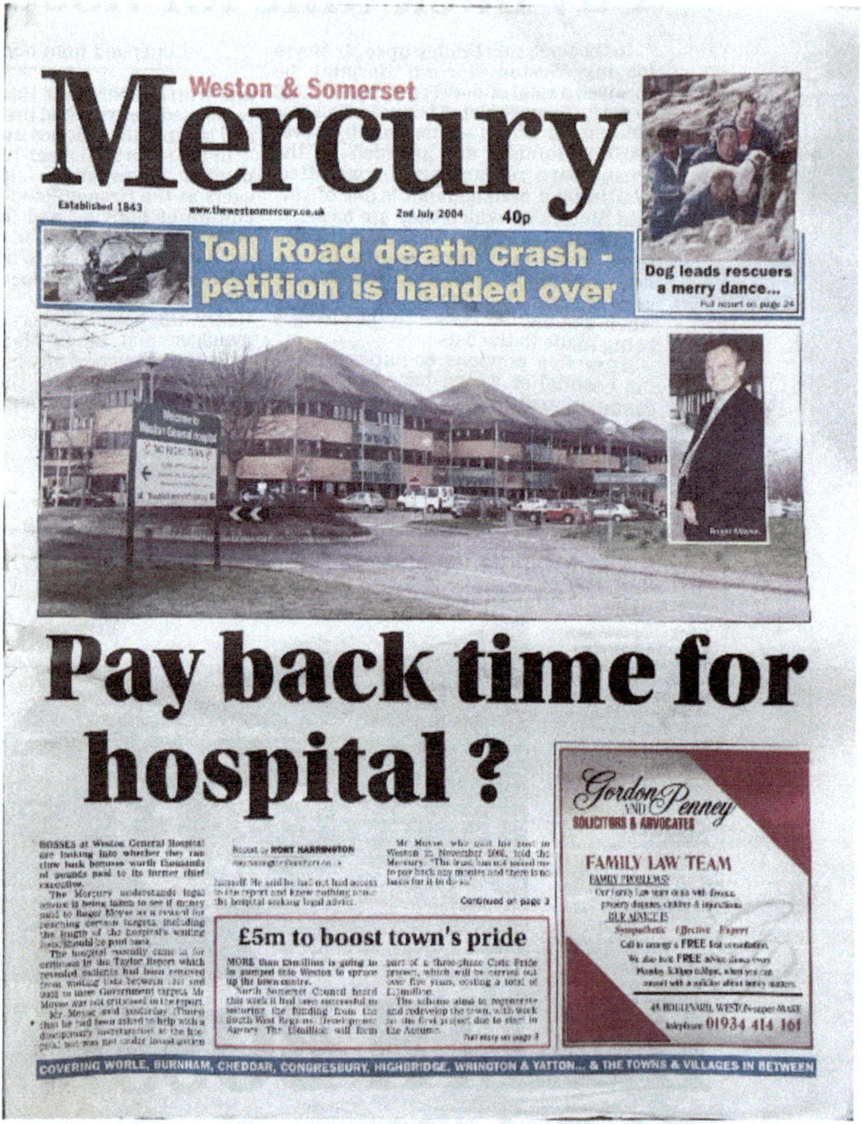

Weston & Somerset

Mercury

Established 1843 www.thewestonmercury.co.uk 2nd July 2004 40p

Toll Road death crash - petition is handed over

Dog leads rescuers a merry dance...

Pay back time for hospital ?

BOSSES at Weston General Hospital are looking into whether they can claw back bonuses worth thousands of pounds paid to its former chief executive.

Continued on page 3

£5m to boost town's pride

COVERING WORLE, BURNHAM, CHEDDAR, CONGRESBURY, HIGHBRIDGE, WRINGTON & YATTON... & THE TOWNS & VILLAGES IN BETWEEN

"Bosses at Weston General are looking into whether they can claw back bonuses worth thousands of pounds paid to the former Chief Executive". Add to this the legal fees for getting me sacked likely to be multiples of his bonus payments. See below!

Pay back time for hospital?

Continued from front page

In the five years leading up to Mr Moyse leaving Weston General Hospital, he received a total of between £28,000-£36,000 in performance-related bonuses. This was paid on top of his annual salary of over £90,000. Bonuses are awarded by the trust board remuneration committee. Waiting list management is one of several factors on which they are based.

The Taylor Report backed up allegations made by former waiting list co-ordinator Michelle Masson, who was suspended from her job in October 2002 when she alerted bosses to the changes being made to the lists.

After five previous enquiries cleared the hospital of wrong-doing, the report, commissioned by Avon, Gloucestershire and Wiltshire Strategic Health Authority, concluded the trust had lied about figures and covered the practice up.

In his report, Michael Taylor, an independent investigator, slammed managers at the Grange Road hospital for a culture of bullying and for using their authority to force junior staff to carry out actions they knew to be wrong.

This week, an independent human resources specialist cleared Marion Henry, the hospital's corporate services manager, and Linda Marvin, the outpatient manager, of any malpractice.

Investigations into the actions of three other people are ongoing.

I was told to fiddle waiting list figures, says whistle-blower

by ANDREW WHITE

SOME senior managers at Weston-super-Mare General Hospital may face disciplinary action and even dismissal after an independent inquiry found they ordered waiting list figures to be fiddled.

The latest investigation, ordered by the Avon, Gloucestershire and Wiltshire Strategic Health Authority, also uncovered bullying in some departments at the hospital in Grange Road, Uphill.

The new inquiry followed persistent claims by Michele Masson, a former waiting list co-ordinator, that she manipulated figures on the instructions of senior management to give the impression that the hospital was meeting Government targets.

▶ Turn to Page 2

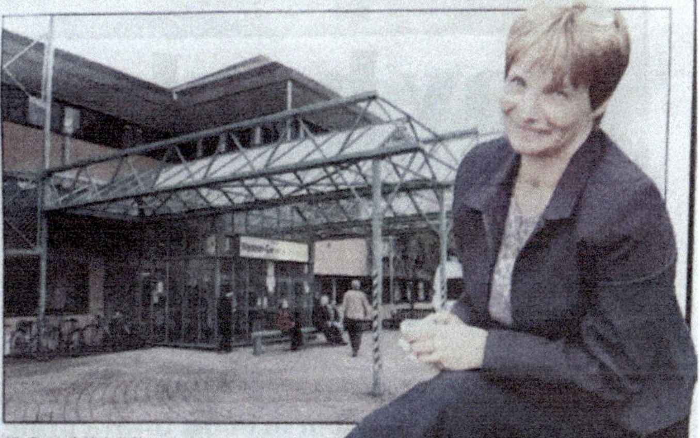

Vindicated: Michele Masson, right, says she was ordered to manipulate waiting list figures at Weston General Hospital, above

HEALTH BOSSES FACE THE SACK

There has been **no accountability** for my suspension and wrongful sacking by Roger Moyse.

Unhealthy position

UNITED Bristol Healthcare Trust and Weston Area Health Trust are in the bottom 30 NHS trusts in the country for the length of time it takes them to refer outpatients.

by SARAH KEY

The trusts were being reviewed as part of a nationwide investigation into hospitals carried out by health watchdog body Dr Foster. There are 153 trusts in England.

UBHT was found to have scored average or above on all other factors looked at by the review panel.

The trust, which runs the Bristol Royal Infirmary and four other hospitals, was found to have a poor 13-week referral rate for outpatients, but did meet the Government target on 17-week referrals to appointment.

Dr Foster was measuring the trust against next year's planned targets, which aim to get patients through to an appointment within 13 weeks.

Robert Woolley, director of performance management at UBHT, said: "The NHS Plan target is that no patient should wait more than 17 weeks for an outpatient appointment, which we have achieved.

"The deadline for a maximum wait of 13 weeks is December 2005, which we are confident we will also achieve.

"The number of our patients waiting up to three months for an outpatient appointment has not decreased over the past year. But, as well as reducing overall outpatient waiting times, we have made significant progress in offering flexible appointment times, with 76 per cent of patients offered an outpatient appointment at a time of their convenience, against a national target of 66 per cent. Our inpatient and day case times are on target."

Weston Area Health Trust, which runs the Weston General Hospital, scored in the lowest 20 trusts in the country for 13-week referrals but met the 17-week referral targets. Mortality rates were higher than last year but the next figures were expected to show improvement.

New chief executive Mark Gritten said: "The trust is looking in depth at the data provided by Dr Foster's report. As a smaller-than-average hospital we are not surprised that there has been a move that might be an expected variation year to year."

s.key@bepp.co.uk

EVENING POST 19.05.04

Hospital chief to quit by end of the year

THE chief executive of Weston Area Health Trust Roger Moyse is expected to leave by the end of the year.

He is thought to be one of the longest-serving health trust chief executives in the country.

The hospital was recently given one star rating in the NHS Performance Ratings.

A trust spokesman said: "There is no question of any financial irregularities at the trust. He thought it was an appropriate time to go having improved the hospital from a zero star rating to a one star rating."

But the latest figures show the hospital would have been £2million in debt over the last financial year had it not sold off the on-site houses used by doctors and nurses to a housing association for £1.8million.

The hospital's finance director Meredith Collins says huge cuts will have to be made during the next financial year in order to balance the books.

Mr Collins said bringing in agency nurses to cope with the number of patients in the hospital accounts for most of the overspend.

The rest of the cash has been spent on treating patients on waiting lists in the private sector.

Mr Collins said a strict financial recovery plan would have to be followed in order for bosses at the hospital to get their heads above water.

"We will be employing more staff to reduce our costs. Agency nurses cost three times more than our own staff," he said.

"By doing this, we will be making sure patients get efficient service and see faces they recognise and trust.

"We will be working with the primary care trust to look at our investments and see how we can save money in the next financial year.

"It is a serious problem, but I do not think it affects the public.

"The changes we are making will benefit patients as they will be getting medical treatment from permanent doctors and nurses."

The hospital's total expenditure for the year was £49million.

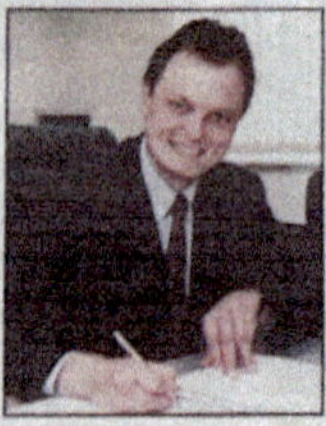

▲ Roger Moyse

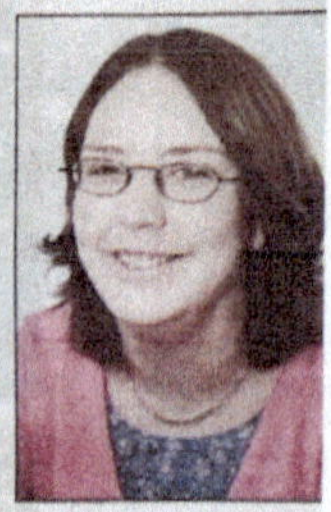

Meet our new

This mission statement "***To ensure the services provided by the Trust meet all relevant standards***" is *laughable* given the protected disclosures I made to the SHA.

14th May 2004 WESTON & SOMERSET MERCURY

Hospital waiting lists were fiddled - official

IN AN astonishing U-turn, Weston General Hospital has admitted that it fiddled patient waiting lists to meet Government targets.

Report by **RORY HARRINGTON**
rory.harrington@archant.co.uk

The damaging admission came as an independent report was made public which showed patients had been removed from the waiting lists between 1999 and 2002.

The changes were made so that when the figures were given to Avon Health Authority, the lists appeared to be shorter than they actually were.

Five previous inquiries, three internal and two external, had all cleared Weston Area Health Trust of lying about the figures and covering the practice up.

But the latest investigation, commissioned by the Avon, Gloucestershire and Wiltshire Strategic Health Authority and called the Taylor Report, also criticised a culture of "heavy handed pressure and bullying" by senior managers against some junior staff at the hospital.

At this time Roger Moyse was the chief executive at the hospital. He left the hospital in November last year after Weston General was awarded one star in hospital league tables.

Mr Moyse earned over £95,000 a year at the hospital.

Weston Area Health Trust chief executive Mark Gritten said there was evidence that senior managers, from director level downwards, had directly falsified the information on waiting lists and used their authority to force junior staff to carry out actions they knew to be wrong.

Mr Gritten confirmed an inquiry will be launched. A small number of senior managers are to be investigated and may face the sack as a result of the scandal.

The report backs up the whistleblowing allegations of former waiting list co-ordinator, Michele Masson, who was suspended from her job in October 2002 after alerting bosses to the deception.

She said: "The first inquiry in 2003 was undoubtedly a cover-up and I hope other members of staff will feel confident of speaking up without fear of consequences."

Mr Gritten said: "We accept the findings and recommendations of the Taylor Report and I apologise to our patients and our local community in Weston.

"I have also apologised to Michele Masson."

In order to tackle the bullying culture that has existed in the Grange Road hospital, chiefs are considering the introduction of a football-style yellow card system.

Staff who feel they are being browbeaten by bosses or colleagues could hold up a yellow card as a warning.

● Further criticism has been levelled at the hospital this week when it was revealed the bill for temporary nursing staff leapt from nearly £83,000 in 1997 to over £2million in 2003 - a 27-fold increase.

Mark Gritten explained this had happened across the whole NHS as the pressure to increase the number of beds had to be matched by more nurses.

While more nurses were being trained, agency staff have been used to cover the shortfall.

The number of agency staff is now falling as more trained nurses come through and Mr Gritten said he expected the hospital bill for temporary nurses to drop to £1.4million in 2004.

An internal report published this week also slammed cleanliness in the hospital as contributing to the recent Norwalk virus outbreak.

Hospital bosses hope replacing ageing bed pan washers and providing an extra £50,000 funding will prevent further outbreaks.

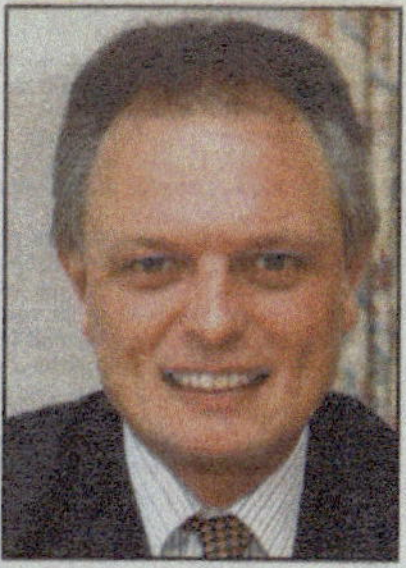

▲ Roger Moyse, former chief executive at Weston General Hospital.

Bosses vindicated after inquiry into manipulation of figures

Waiting list fiddle: top staff cleared

TWO senior staff members at Weston General Hospital have been cleared of any involvement with fiddling the hospital's waiting lists.

However, inquiries are continuing into the conduct and performance of other members of staff at the hospital.

It is believed that three people are still being investigated and could face possible disciplinary action.

The results of an independent inquiry by NHS investigator Michael Taylor announced in May supported claims by former waiting list co-ordinator Michele Masson that figures were manipulated.

Mrs Masson alleged that the figures were adjusted on the instructions of senior management to give the impression that the hospital was meeting government targets.

But an independent adviser to the Weston Area Health Trust in the wake of the Taylor Report has now found there was no evidence to suggest that corporate services manager Marion Henry and out-patient manager Linda Marvin were in any way involved with the malpractice.

In fact, he commended the pair for their efforts in endeavouring to ensure that a thorough investigation was carried out.

A statement issued by the WAHT says: "The trust acknowledges that at the time, the management structure and span of control in this area of the trust's operations was untenable.

"It also recognises that the handling of the original allegations has placed a significant strain on trust staff, including Linda Marvin and Marion Henry."

Meanwhile, the trust confirmed investigations into the conduct and performance of other members of staff are continuing.

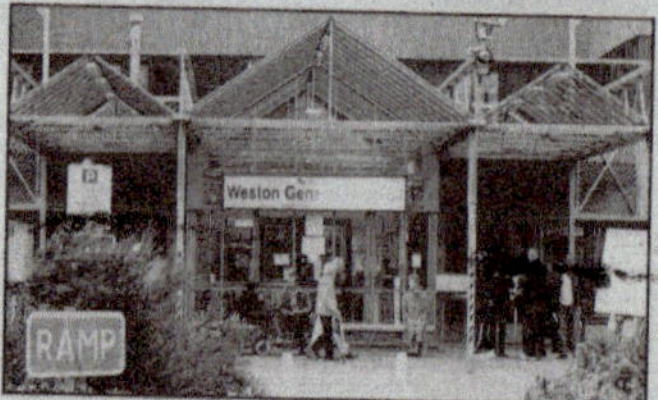

Inquiry: Weston General Hospital, where two senior members of staff have been cleared of fiddling waiting lists

by ANDREW WHITE

When the results of the Taylor Report were announced, the WAHT chief executive, Mark Gritten, said some senior managers could be dismissed if they were found to be fiddling waiting lists.

Mr Taylor found that most of Mrs Masson's claims were true and that between 1999 and 2002, patient data was deliberately held back from the active waiting list, there was the inappropriate deferral of patients from waiting lists and a failure to remove patients from waiting lists when they no longer needed treatment.

a.white@bepp.co.uk

12 WESTON AREA HEALTH TRUST ANNUAL REPORT 2001/2002

The Trust's mission statement

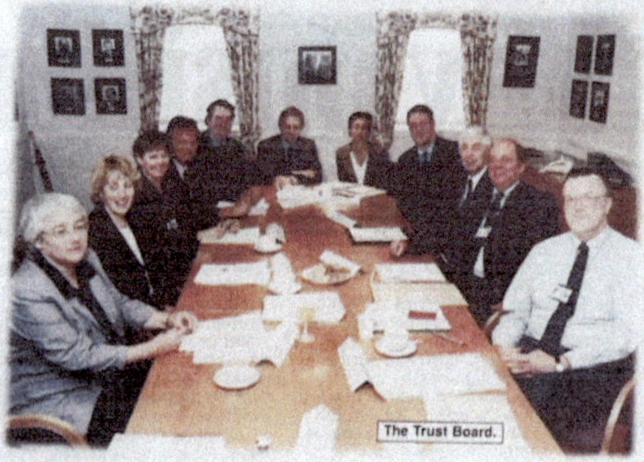

The Trust Board.

- To provide high quality local healthcare services

OBJECTIVES OF THE TRUST:

- To provide a caring, responsive and co-ordinated hospital and community service to a high quality for the local population
- To ensure that close integration exists between acute (hospital) and community services and to generate close working relationships with the General Practitioners in Weston and the surrounding area
- To ensure that the services provided by the Trust meet all relevant standards
- To provide job satisfaction for staff and meet their personal and career development needs
- To develop teaching and training for medical, nursing and other health service staff
- To ensure that a co-operative and supporting working relationship exists with the League of Friends, volunteer workers and voluntary bodies
- As an integral part of the NHS, to maximise our effectiveness
- To involve the local population in decisions about the services provided by the Trust

Looking back at the year gives no mention of the fact I was sacked, or why I raised concerns.

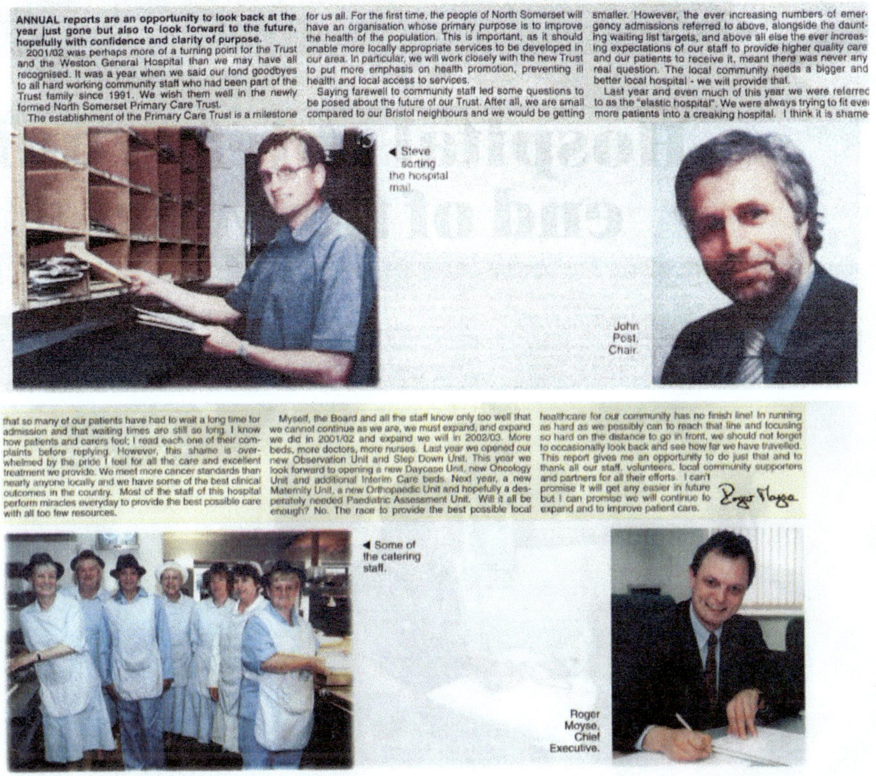

ANNUAL reports are an opportunity to look back at the year just gone but also to look forward to the future, hopefully with confidence and clarity of purpose.

2001/02 was perhaps more of a turning point for the Trust and the Weston General Hospital than we may have all recognised. It was a year when we said our fond goodbyes to all hard working community staff who had been part of the Trust family since 1991. We wish them well in the newly formed North Somerset Primary Care Trust.

The establishment of the Primary Care Trust is a milestone for us all. For the first time, the people of North Somerset will have an organisation whose primary purpose is to improve the health of the population. This is important, as it should enable more locally appropriate services to be developed in our area. In particular, we will work closely with the new Trust to put more emphasis on health promotion, preventing ill health and local access to services.

Saying farewell to community staff led some questions to be posed about the future of our Trust. After all, we are small compared to our Bristol neighbours and we would be getting smaller. However, the ever increasing numbers of emergency admissions referred to above, alongside the daunting waiting list targets, and above all else the ever increasing expectations of our staff to provide higher quality care and our patients to receive it, meant there was never any real question. The local community needs a bigger and better local hospital - we will provide that.

Last year and even much of this year we were referred to as the "elastic hospital". We were always trying to fit ever more patients into a creaking hospital. I think it is shameful that so many of our patients have had to wait a long time for admission and that waiting times are still so long. I know how patients and carers feel; I read each one of their complaints before replying. However, this shame is overwhelmed by the pride I feel for all the care and excellent treatment we provide. We meet more cancer standards than nearly anyone locally and we have some of the best clinical outcomes in the country. Most of the staff of this hospital perform miracles everyday to provide the best possible care with all too few resources.

Myself, the Board and all the staff know only too well that we cannot continue as we are, we must expand, and expand we did in 2001/02 and expand we will in 2002/03. More beds, more doctors, more nurses. Last year we opened our new Observation Unit and Step Down Unit. This year we look forward to opening a new Daycase Unit, new Oncology Unit and additional Interim Care beds. Next year, a new Maternity Unit, a new Orthopaedic Unit and hopefully a desperately needed Paediatric Assessment Unit. Will it all be enough? No. The race to provide the best possible local healthcare for our community has no finish line! In running as hard as we possibly can to reach that line and focusing so hard on the distance to go in front, we should not forget to occasionally look back and see how far we have travelled. This report gives me an opportunity to do just that and to thank all our staff, volunteers, local community supporters and partners for all their efforts. I can't promise it will get any easier in future but I can promise we will continue to expand and to improve patient care.

◀ Steve sorting the hospital mail.

John Post, Chair.

◀ Some of the catering staff.

Roger Moyse, Chief Executive.

Chief Executive Roger Moyse - quote "*I know how patients and carers feel; I read each one of their complaints before replying*". Yet not one of the concerns I raised in writing was given a response in the seven months before I was suspended or since. I believe I made protected disclosures and was a whistleblower as is typical in these situations. The trust's view that the reason they gave for your dismissal was *the 'irretrievable breakdown of trust and confidence'*. However, this differed from the agreed statement. I felt bullied, undermined and wrongly deemed incompetent. I was referred to occupational health and the consultant, no surprise to me, said he found no problems with my mental health. Then followed the investigation with the NCAA and despite the NCAA deeming me competent, the Trust referred me to the GMC, who did not see any need to investigate me.

Weston & Somerset Mercury

Issue No.7674 www.thewestonmercury.co.uk Established 1843 January 3rd 2003 35p

Heart specialist is sacked by hospital

A TOP consultant has been dismissed from Weston General Hospital after a catalogue of complaints from colleagues.

Dr Lance Forbat was employed as a consultant physician with the Trust in January 2002 and specialised in cardiology.

But after just seven months at the hospital Dr Forbat was suspended after a number of concerns about his professional behaviour.

The decision was taken after complaints were received from doctors, nurses and technicians.

A statement from Weston Area Health Trust said: "Staff complained that Dr Forbat failed to prioritise the basic duties of an NHS consultant, failed to give clear guidance to junior colleagues and was generally disorganised."

In view of these complaints the Trust has now officially dismissed Dr Forbat.

Reports on Dr Forbat's dismissal will now be sent to the General Medical Council to ensure a proper investigation.

Page 14 Mid Somerset Newspapers January 9, 2003

Multi-million pound treatment centre opens

By Oliver Hulme

A £3 million treatment centre to serve out-patients from the Cheddar Valley area and perform routine operations opened at Weston General Hospital on Monday.

The Day Case Unit – so called because treatment is completed in one day and should not require an overnight stay – has been built within the hospital's Jackson Barstow wing and contains a state-of-the-art centre for ear, nose and throat treatments, orthopaedics, and oral/dental and general surgery.

Doctors at the unit will treat patients under both general and local anaesthetic.

There are two operating theatres and the unit will treat up to 6,000 people a year from the area, including the Cheddar Valley.

Roger Moyse, chief executive of Weston Area Health Trust, said: "The new Day Case Unit will bring great benefits to our patients.

"They will be able to book an appointment that is convenient to them, have their necessary surgery and be home in time for tea.

"We will be able to see more people more quickly, which can only mean good news for local residents."

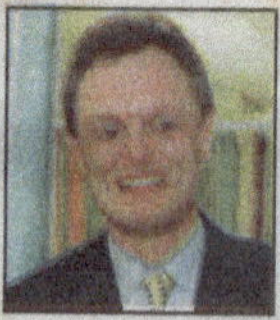

Chief executive of Weston Area Health Trust Roger Moyse

The unit has been designed to use the latest technology, with everything from surgical equipment to a "circular track" system to make it easy for patients to get from reception to treatment and into the recovery room with ease.

Even the walls of the consulting room have been painted a colour which will help clinicians see quickly if patients are looking ill.

From March, patients will be able to see their specialist, have their pre-operation assessment and book the date of their operation all on the same day.

The Day Case Unit was built with the help of of Weston General Hospital's League Of Friends, and the Jackson Barstow Wing was built with a bequest from Enid Sybil Jackson Barstow.

Consultant at hospital is sacked

Health chiefs in Weston-super-Mare have sacked a consultant from the general hospital, which covers some of the Cheddar Valley area.

The board of the Weston Area Health NHS Trust has endorsed the decision of chief executive Roger Moyse to dismiss Dr Lance Forbat.

Dr Forbat was a consultant physician with a particular interest in cardiology who was employed by the trust last January, but has not been at work since July after concerns were expressed about his professional behaviour.

A statement issued by the trust said it had become evident there was a breakdown in working relationships with a number of his colleagues.

The trust received a number of complaints from doctors, nurses and technicians working with Dr Forbat.

Staff complained of failure to prioritise the basic duties of an NHS consultant, failure to give clear guidance to junior colleagues and general disorganisation.

The trust now hopes there will be a full investigation into Dr Forbat's clinical competence in the interests of patients.

It intends to send relevant papers to the General Medical Council, which decides whether a doctor is fit to practice.

It is the only authority that can strike a doctor off the medical register.

West Cumberland Times and Star **Friday January 10 2003**

Heart specialist sacked

A DOCTOR hailed as the hero of cardiac patients at the West Cumberland Hospital has been sacked from his job at Weston-Super-Mare General Hospital after just 12 months.

Dr Lance Forbat's sacking was the result of complaints from colleagues about his failure to prioritise basic duties, failure to give clear guidance to junior colleagues and general disorganisation.

The Weston Area Health NHS Trust said it hopes there will be a full investigation into Dr Forbat's clinical competence in the interest of patients.

The doctor's decision to leave West Cumbria for personal reasons in October 2001 was met with dismay by the West Cumbria Heart and Angina Support Group.

The group's founder Ronnie Copeland, said it was probably Dr Forbat's vision and fight for improvements that led to problems in his new post. He said the work he had done was phenomenal.

Whitehaven News
Thursday 16/1/03

Dr Forbat deserves our support

SIR – The sacking of Dr Forbat from his post at Weston-super-Mare General Hospital, (The Whitehaven News, January 9), is quite incredible. How on earth could a consultant whose work in West Cumbria over seven years was so widely acclaimed be found wanting within seven months at another hospital? To ask the General Medical Council to decide whether he is fit to practice seems quite ludicrous in view of his record in our area.

I was referred to Dr Forbat five years ago and found him extremely thorough, requiring a wide range of tests before reaching a conclusion. In my case surgery was not required, but a number of friends who have had heart bypass surgery under his direction found their lives transformed as a result and speak extremely highly of his prodigious energy and care for those who most needed his help.

Certainly Dr Forbat was demanding in his drive for better facilities in our area and he would not have achieved so much had he been less determined. One formed the impression that he was not a man to suffer fools gladly – could it be that he found them in Weston-super-Mare?

West Cumbria should support Dr Forbat at this time, both to ensure that a balanced view of his work is seen by the General Medical Council and so that he is personally aware of the appreciation of his former patients in this area. Should we not also explore the possibility of enticing him back to West Cumbria where he would be appreciated and could continue the work he started here?

Michael FORSDYKE
Wilton
Egremont

P.S. Nothing in Times and Star or Cumberland News.

Bulling in the Trust led to the resignation of the first wholetime consultant haematologist appointed 2005, Dr Frank Booth. He was trying to attain the standards of the national regulatory bodies. He explains why he left in 2010 in his letter of 23 June 2011 to the Weston and Somerset Mercury.

23rd June, 2011 WESTON & SOMERSET MERCURY www.westonmercury.co.uk 61

Consultant: 'Why I left the Weston hospital trust'

I AM writing to explain to the people of Weston and its surroundings the circumstances that led to me leaving Weston Area Health NHS Trust, where I worked as a consultant haematologist from 2005 until August 2010.

They will otherwise never know the reasons for my departure as the trust will certainly never make these public.

The formal explanation will simply be that I retired, which is technically true but belies the facts of the matter.

I have lived with and worked for the NHS all of my life. I cherish it and have worked long and hard to sustain it in some small way throughout my career in medicine.

I have seen many changes in the 35 years since I qualified but I have always taken the view, as do many of us who work in the NHS, that I am a public servant and ultimately accountable to the public who fund the service.

There have been difficult times when the only important criterion for Trust chief executives was to balance the books at the end of the year.

This ended when clinical governance came to the fore. Quality of care became an issue of equal importance and regulatory bodies were set up to define standards and monitor adherence to these. Regretfully, it is sometimes too easy for hospitals to pay lip service to some of these standards and to compromise patient care as a consequence.

Having seen this happen too often in the past (I worked as a consultant in three other trusts before I came to Weston), I have taken a particular interest in clinical governance and in analysing clinical systems to assess what makes them work well and also why failures occur, as they inevitably will from time to time, even in the best regulated organisations.

Failures can occur as a result of individual shortcomings or genuine errors and will do so whenever humans are involved in the process.

Clearly, it is important to have appropriately trained staff and the right skill mix to run the service but the staff must also be appropriately supported to make effective contributions to any system in which they work.

Badly designed and operated systems will inevitably fail more easily and more often and it is the responsibility of trust managers to ensure that the systems for which they are responsible operate effectively and, above all, safely as well as cost effectively. This is always a challenge.

I have never known a time when NHS staff have not claimed that it is underfunded, but the balance has not always been as favourable as it has been in recent years, although clearly we have now entered a new era of austerity.

It is for managers to strike an appropriate balance and to justify expenditure needed to provide safe and effective services for the public, but it is incumbent on those managers to heed the advice of the clinical staff charged with delivering the clinical care. Do not expect them to provide safe care with inadequate resources. Ensure that essential services are safe as well as cost effective. If you cannot achieve all that you might like, at least don't cause harm.

It was against this background that I came to Weston Area Health NHS Trust, the first whole-time consultant haematologist to be employed there.

Hitherto, the clinical haematology service had been provided by visiting consultants from Bristol and the laboratory had very little clinical supervision. Systems vulnerable to error.

I set about trying to attain the standards of clinical laboratory and patient care to which I had been trained to aspire.

Not my standards but those of national regulatory bodies.

I have never shirked work and I put a great deal of effort into making the changes that were needed, with some initial success.

I believe that I helped to transform the clinical haematology service but in the laboratory I was less successful. I was frustrated and dismayed by some of the most senior managers' decisions but was powerless to rectify the situation.

Although nominally the 'clinical lead for haematology', I had no management authority myself and was eventually reduced to pointing out when errors occurred, as they did with alarming frequency, to illustrate where and why the systems were failing.

This did not make me popular with my senior managerial colleagues and I was seen as a nuisance and disloyal. Nothing could have been further from the truth. I lived and worked in Weston, where I was potentially as dependent upon the local healthcare provision as anybody else.

It mattered to me to make sure that we were delivering a safe service and I did my best to ensure that my own contribution was the best that I could manage.

For the most part I believe that the patients under my direct care appreciated my efforts.

I didn't always please everybody but even those who might have preferred to see somebody else can be assured that I always tried my best for every patient who I saw.

By the start of 2010, my own workload had increased to a level that was difficult to manage. At 58 years old I could not sustain excessive working hours indefinitely.

I tried hard to negotiate a reduction to a standard working week, which should have been feasible but was in practice impossible without additional support and, as usual, no funding was available to employ new clinical staff.

I suggested a number of cost-neutral options, all of which were rejected without serious consideration by my managers.

All very frustrating. So I put forward one final suggestion, that I should retire (thereby taking my pension, which appeared under threat with a general election looming).

This would free my entire salary for reinvestment in the service, I hoped to continue to work in a less well paid, perhaps part-time capacity so that we could employ an additional consultant and, overall, provide a sustainable clinical service.

I still had serious reservations about the laboratory but felt that the only way to improve this would eventually be from within. I need not have worried.

I gave five months notice of my intention to retire and my wish to continue as outlined" but, to this day, I have not even been dignified by a response from the trust chief executive.

No post for which I could apply was advertised and so I was obliged to look for work elsewhere. I am now employed as a consultant haematologist on the Isle of Wight.

When, eventually, a consultant post was advertised, in December 2010, nine months after my decision to retire, I applied out of interest.

To my deep regret, but perhaps I should not have been surprised, my application was rejected without further consideration. I was not even offered an interview.

No appointment was made because there were no other suitable applicants and the clinical haematology service has continued to be run by a succession of locums.

So I enquired why I had been rejected out of hand and was informed that 'the trust's decision was informed by the knowledge that during your employment with the trust you maintained difficult working relationships with some trust colleagues'.

I should make it clear that no action has ever been taken against me by the trust. Nor could any have been because my 'crime' has been to point out flawed services.

I have always endeavoured to provide the best service possible in compliance with clinical governance standards.

Unfortunately, some senior managers appear to make up the standards as they go along and they do so with apparent impunity.

Nobody holds them accountable and decisions may be intimidating to the extent that individuals may fear for their jobs.

I have been around some of these people long enough not to be intimidated by them but that makes me a threat and, however well-intentioned I may have been, there is little that I can do about the situation other than make it more widely known and to registered my opinion that this constitutes an abuse of the authority invested in these people by the public of this country and it always represents a threat to patient care.

I can only apologise to the patients for whom I cared and who may feel that I abandoned them.

The official trust line remains that I retired and left of my own volition.

The truth of the matter is that the trust senior managers placed me under great duress and were then happy to abandon me and cover up the service failures. I tried.

DR FRANK BOOTH
Jubilee Place, Cowes, Isle of Wight

Trust Chair John Post at the board meetings had the opportunity, and should have with other non-executive members, taken my concerns seriously and question a. why no attempts were made to respond to me directly? b. why I raised them. In doing so he was complicit in burying the truth because he was more concerned about the reputation of the institution (Charter) than patient safety. By wrongly accusing me of incompetence and referring me to the NCAA they were "*shooting the messenger*".

I subsequently raised these issues in my evidence to the Francis Inquiry. This was the theme that came out in his report and is common to inquiries decade after decade. Here are examples of some before the latest major scandal of the Letby inquiry.

1. **Mid Staffordshire NHS Foundation Trust**: A scandal occurred at Mid Staffordshire NHS Foundation Trust between **2005 and 2009**, where systemic failures in care led to significant harm and unnecessary deaths of patients. A public inquiry, known as the Francis Inquiry, was conducted in **2010–2013** to investigate the deficiencies and recommend improvements to patient safety and care standards.
2. **Morecambe Bay maternity scandal**: In this scandal, it was revealed that poor care at the University Hospitals of Morecambe Bay NHS Foundation Trust led to the deaths of at least 11 babies and one mother between **2004 and 2013**. Investigations and inquiries were held to uncover the failings and improve safety measures.
3. **Shrewsbury and Telford Hospital maternity scandal**: Investigations were launched into maternity services at Shrewsbury and Telford Hospital NHS Trust following numerous reports of poor care, avoidable deaths, and birth injuries to mothers and babies. The scandal, dating back to **1979**, came to light in **2017** and ongoing investigations aim to uncover the extent of the failures.
4. **East Kent maternity scandal**: In **2019**, a BBC investigation shed light on multiple baby deaths at East Kent Hospitals University NHS Foundation Trust. Subsequently, an independent review was launched to examine the maternity services and determine the extent of the failings.
5. **Nottingham maternity investigation 2023**. At the time of writing it has been one year since Ms Ockenden's review into Nottingham University Hospitals' maternity services began. The inquiry is reviewing cases where mothers or babies have died or suffered harm at Nottingham City Hospital and Queen's Medical Centre since 2012. It is expected to become the largest maternity

> inquiry carried out in the UK, with around 1,700 families contacted so far.
>
> The early press release was not shown to me in advance, and I believe was clearly intended to defame me and ruin my reputation. *There was an early release that the BMA wrote formally complaining to the Trust chairman and it was published in several papers in Somerset and Cumbria.* It follows the typical treatment of outspoken caring doctors following whistleblowing. *It felt one-sided and was premature to the NCAA report, GMC decision not to investigate and the later agreed statement. This is why I believe that changes are necessary; to PIDA and the setting up of the Office of the Whistleblower is essential to protect doctors (or other employees) and in the NHS context potentially protect patients, from preventable harm.*

The cost to the taxpayer for my case will have included the Trust's legal fees and subsequent need for locums, as it took some years to recruit a replacement locum cardiologist and longer for the first substantive consultant who decided after only a year to leave for better pastures for a Trust in a nearby county.

The statement released to the press was agreed after representations to the High Court by the Medical Protection Society in an attempt to get me proper compensation, but I was advised not to pursue the case as there was concern about the risk of losing, as the opinion was PIDA was ineffectual. I hoped to avoid the Trust referring me to the GMC, but they did anyway despite the NCAA stating they had no concerns about my clinical ability. The GMC reviewed all the submissions from both parties and then with the NCAA concluded there was no reason to take further action.'

Michael Taylor of NHS Confederation's National Panel of Investigators said there was a culture of "***heavy-handed pressure and bullying***" against certain groups of staff. Mrs Mason, who exposed the waiting list fiddle, received an apology from the new Chief Executive Mark Gritten and Chairman Ron Ballentine "***for the way in which the earlier investigation was carried out***" and to patients and community "***the previous inquiry was flawed.***"

April 2004

STATEMENT

The Trust and Dr. Forbat are pleased to announce that they have settled their differences.

The Trust was pleased to be advised by the NCAA in March 2003 that Dr. Forbat is a competent clinician and noted that the workload in the department was too much for a single-handed consultant. Furthermore, the General Medical Council, to whom the Trust referred matters, decided in Summer 2003 that it did not need to take any action.

The Trust has appointed 2 consultants to replace Dr. Forbat and has apologised to Dr. Forbat for its treatment of him and agreed to pay him damages.

Both Dr. Forbat and the Trust hope that, now that they have resolved their differences, it will be possible for all concerned to put these matters behind them.

NEWS Thursday, May 13 2004

Hospital bosses' pledge over waiting lists

▶ From Page 1

It followed an earlier inquiry by a specialist management consultancy that advises the National Health Service on personnel issues which, last year cleared senior Weston Area Health Trust (WAHT) staff of any wrongdoing.

The latest inquiry was conducted by Michael Taylor, of the NHS Confederation's National Panel of Investigators, who concluded that most of Mrs Masson's allegations were true.

He found that between 1999 and 2002 there was:

- Deliberate holding back of patient data from the active waiting list
- Inappropriate deferral of patients from the in-patient waiting list
- A failure to remove patients from waiting lists when it was clear they no longer needed treatment

But he was not able to find conclusively that there was an inappropriate deferral of patients from the out-patient waiting list.

Mr Taylor also decided that Mrs Masson was "complicit in condoning inappropriate practices" and was at fault for not exposing the concern of her staff until it suited her personally.

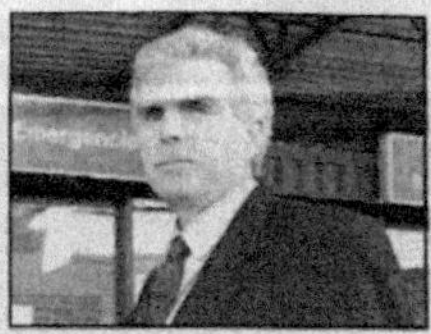

Issued apology: Mark Gritten, WAHT's new chief executive

But he felt that this was partly due to the fact that she had received direct instructions from her superiors to manipulate figures and said that a culture of "heavy handed pressure and bullying" against certain groups of staff had developed at the trust.

Mr Taylor found the allegation by Mrs Masson that a number of patients who may have been deferred before 1999 were never reported on the waiting list was invalid.

He decided that the basic reason why the earlier inquiry did not get to the truth of the matter was because it focused on Mrs Masson leaving the trust.

Mrs Masson, aged 48, was suspended from duty in October 2002 and resigned two months later. She now lives in Spain but returned to Weston yesterday for the announcement of Mr Taylor findings.

She met the WAHT's new chief executive, Mark Gritten and new chairman Ron Ballantine.

The two men apologised to her for the way in which the earlier investigation was carried out.

Mr Gritten, who also apologised to patients and the community, accepted the previous inquiry was flawed. He said: "Clearly, her allegations were not fully and robustly investigated.

"Formal investigations into the conduct and performance of individuals has started and is likely to lead to disciplinary action which could result in dismissal."

Mr Gritten said the full contents of Mr Taylor's report could not be published at this time for legal and disciplinary reasons.

He said: "I would like to stress that it is only a handful of staff involved in this and a small number of patients. The report says the vast majority of staff are hard working and dedicated and care passionately about providing a good service for the community."

Mr Gritten gave an assurance that the waiting list figures were now accurate said he was working to create a better atmosphere at the hospital so that staff were not afraid to voice any concerns.

Speaking outside the hospital before returning to Spain, Mrs Masson said: "I feel relieved and vindicated."

"I hope other members of the NHS will feel more confident about speaking up."

Mrs Masson was concerned that some patients may have been adversely affected by what had happened and could now consider taking appropriate action.

She said the first inquiry, ordered by the then WAHT chief executive Roger Moyse, who resigned suddenly towards the end of last year, was a "cover up."

And she questioned whether some other senior management figures at the hospital should remain in their jobs or even within the NHS.

a.white@bepp.co.uk

There was no lacking in bad publicity for Weston General Hospital after I left. I had to sit back and watch as my whistleblowing was buried in the archives of the Trust. Attempts to merge with Musgrove Park Hospital had been planned when I was there but failed to materialise. The irony is eventually Weston General joined the Bristol flagship hospital BRI, which was the source of the original Bristol Baby scandal that in the sacking of the anaesthetist Stephen Bolsin who raised concerns about baby deaths and following the publication of the Kennedy report, before my imminent arrival at Weston!

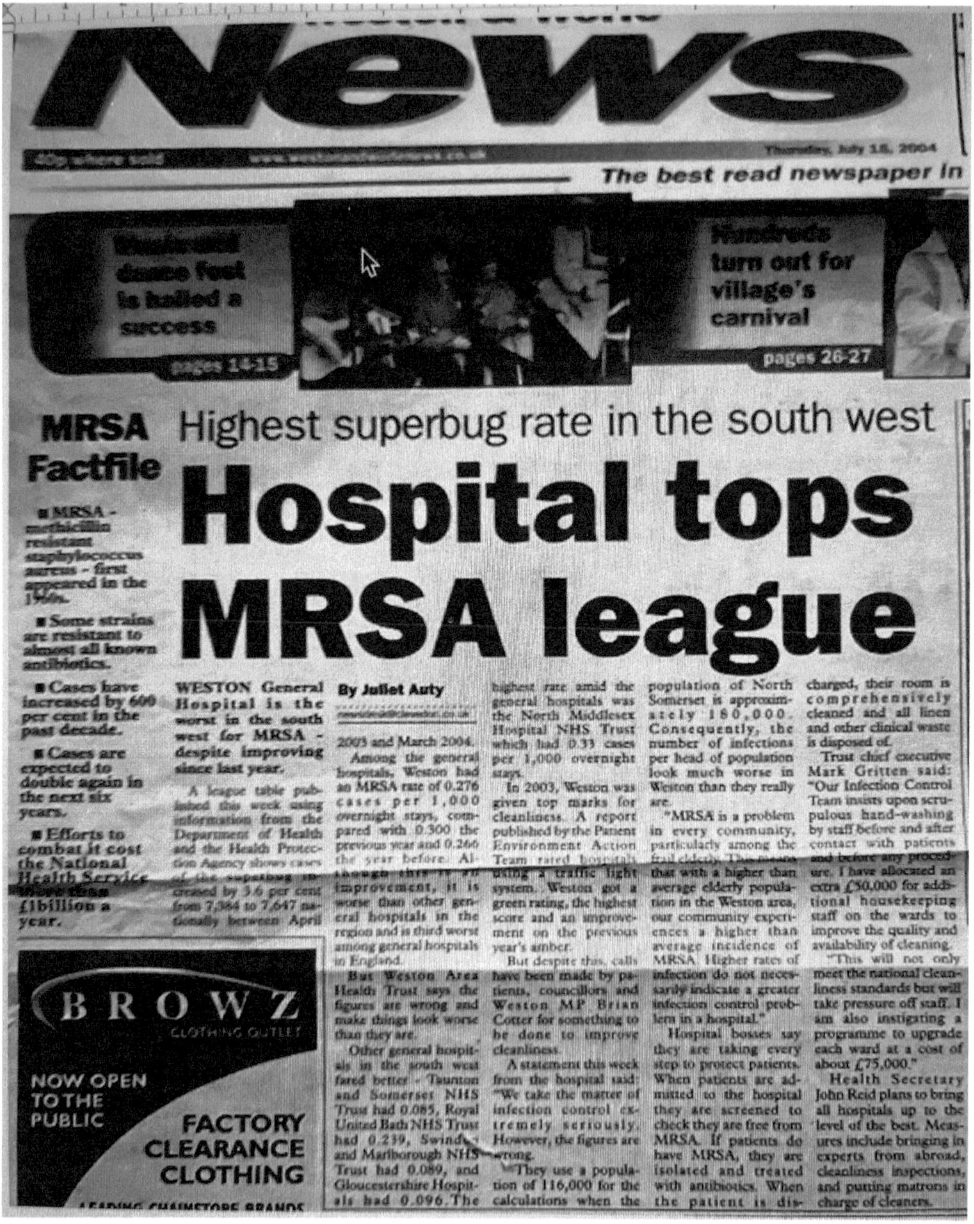

News

Thursday, July 15, 2004

The best read newspaper in

dance fest is hailed a success

pages 14-15

Hundreds turn out for village's carnival

pages 26-27

MRSA Factfile

- MRSA - methicillin resistant staphylococcus aureus - first appeared in the 1960s.
- Some strains are resistant to almost all known antibiotics.
- Cases have increased by 600 per cent in the past decade.
- Cases are expected to double again in the next six years.
- Efforts to combat it cost the National Health Service more than £1billion a year.

Highest superbug rate in the south west

Hospital tops MRSA league

WESTON General Hospital is the worst in the south west for MRSA - despite improving since last year.

By Juliet Auty

A league table published this week using information from the Department of Health and the Health Protection Agency shows cases of the superbug increased by 3.6 per cent from 7,384 to 7,647 nationally between April 2003 and March 2004.

Among the general hospitals, Weston had an MRSA rate of 0.276 cases per 1,000 overnight stays, compared with 0.300 the previous year and 0.266 the year before. Although this is an improvement, it is worse than other general hospitals in the region and is third worst among general hospitals in England.

But Weston Area Health Trust says the figures are wrong and make things look worse than they are.

Other general hospitals in the south west fared better - Taunton and Somerset NHS Trust had 0.085, Royal United Bath NHS Trust had 0.239, Swindon and Marlborough NHS Trust had 0.089, and Gloucestershire Hospitals had 0.096. The highest rate amid the general hospitals was the North Middlesex Hospital NHS Trust which had 0.33 cases per 1,000 overnight stays.

In 2003, Weston was given top marks for cleanliness. A report published by the Patient Environment Action Team rated hospitals using a traffic light system. Weston got a green rating, the highest score and an improvement on the previous year's amber.

But despite this, calls have been made by patients, councillors and Weston MP Brian Cotter for something to be done to improve cleanliness.

A statement this week from the hospital said: "We take the matter of infection control extremely seriously. However, the figures are wrong.

"They use a population of 116,000 for the calculations when the population of North Somerset is approximately 180,000. Consequently, the number of infections per head of population look much worse in Weston than they really are.

"MRSA is a problem in every community, particularly among the frail elderly. This means that with a higher than average elderly population in the Weston area, our community experiences a higher than average incidence of MRSA. Higher rates of infection do not necessarily indicate a greater infection control problem in a hospital."

Hospital bosses say they are taking every step to protect patients. When patients are admitted to the hospital they are screened to check they are free from MRSA. If patients do have MRSA, they are isolated and treated with antibiotics. When the patient is discharged, their room is comprehensively cleaned and all linen and other clinical waste is disposed of.

Trust chief executive Mark Gritten said: "Our Infection Control Team insists upon scrupulous hand-washing by staff before and after contact with patients and before any procedure. I have allocated an extra £50,000 for additional housekeeping staff on the wards to improve the quality and availability of cleaning.

"This will not only meet the national cleanliness standards but will take pressure off staff. I am also instigating a programme to upgrade each ward at a cost of about £75,000."

Health Secretary John Reid plans to bring all hospitals up to the level of the best. Measures include bringing in experts from abroad, cleanliness inspections, and putting matrons in charge of cleaners.

Poor performers wait 30 weeks for NCAA assessment

SUSPENSIONS

POORLY-PERFORMING doctors are having to wait as long as seven months for the results of investigations by the body aimed at reducing suspensions.

The process, undertaken by the National Clinical Assessment Authority, is taking up to four months longer than planned.

Doctors referred to the body are assessed by a team which examines behavioural, clinical and health influences and any other factors that may affect the doctor's work. This information forms the basis of a report which is used to outline an action plan. This may involve the doctor participating in a re-education programme or mentoring system.

The delays have largely been attributed to the lack of medical assessors, but are much longer than the authority's three-month aim.

Its medical director, Dr Alastair Scotland, said once the target of 70 assessors had been recruited, the process would be completed a lot faster.

'One of the biggest factors in cases being delayed is getting access to assessors, which is not surprising because, at the moment, we are very much working on the goodwill of people because we haven't got our own panel.'

He said another contributory factor was that the assessments had been a lot more complex than anticipated.

The lack of assessors means the authority will not meet its target for 80 per cent of cases to be handled within 84 days.

Dr Peter Tomlin, secretary of the suspensions study group of the Society of Clinical Psychiatrists, said the waiting time was 'far too long', and many cases where doctors were proved to be incompetent could have been proved within weeks.

'When we have looked at cases done in the past, they scream out [that] they could have been sorted out within three or four weeks.'

But he did believe a delay could be expected if a specialist was being assessed in terms of competence, as it could take time to put a team together.

Dr Scotland said the nature of the NCAA's expected work had changed from a 'simple' assessment or advice service, to a more complicated process of working through to see if an assessment was necessary.

News in brief

Investigations fall

The number of doctors being referred to the NCAA has dropped by more than a quarter. Of the 268 cases brought to its attention in the first nine months of the 2002-03 financial year, 173 came from hospitals and 95 involved GPs. The figure is lower than the 362 referrals the body was expecting. Dr Alastair Scotland, its medical director, said the lower caseload meant the authority was dealing with fewer complicated cases. He believed this could change as more doctors became aware of the NCAA's work.

Education drive

The NCAA is to launch a series of initiatives to tackle poor performance. An education programme is the next major step for the organisation, which has so far concentrated on assessments of doctors with difficulties. It is also launching an Internet database to provide information on NHS policies and give trusts the opportunity to share ideas and examples of good working practice. An NCAA spokeswoman said: 'We've always said our role is to help the NHS, and this is a key tool in achieving that.'

Weston-super-Mare

Health care in North Somerset is among the worst in

Good news and bad as the NHS gets exam marks

By Chris Roe and Nick Pearson
wdnews@bepp.co.uk

HEALTH care in North Somerset will come under harsh scrutiny today as the area's two main NHS organisations are ranked among the worst in the country.

Both Weston Area Health Trust and North Somerset Primary Care Trust failed to score a single ratings star between them. Their performance sticks out in the West, where standards were otherwise among the UK's best.

Bosses at both trusts were quick to claim that the real picture is much less bleak than the official figures suggest.

Elsewhere in the Bristol area things were looking up for the city's larger trusts, which both gained crucial stars.

But Mark Gritten, chief executive of the area health trust which runs Weston General Hospital, said yesterday the situation had improved "dramatically" since his arrival in January and figures covering the whole of 2003-04 did not reflect that. Vital targets, such as cancer treatment waiting times and hospital cleanliness, had also been met.

The hospital, which achieved a single star last year, fell down over a £1.5million overspend and a narrow miss on the target to treat accident and emergency patients within four hours.

"As a relatively small trust that experienced its busiest ever year last year we have much to be proud of, and I am confident that this will be reflected next year," said Mr Gritten.

Julie Sharma, North Somerset PCT chief executive, said: "I am very disappointed by this rating. It masks the tremendous work undertaken by our staff throughout a year that has led to many service improvements for our population."

She said that eight out of nine key targets were now being met and the trust would work with other bodies to improve its performance. It had also been penalised for not achieving financial balance, a situation partly caused by an unexpected rise in emergency admissions.

"We should not lose sight of the fact that our patients believe that the NHS locally does a good job," she said. "Thousands of patients are seen in our hospitals, by family doctors or in the community each and every day and receive an ever increasing standard of care."

In Bristol the news was better.

North Bristol NHS Trust, which runs Southmead and Frenchay hospitals, regained the one star it lost last year.

However, the commission made it clear there was still work to be done - passing it on only seven of the nine key target areas.

But it was at the United Bristol Healthcare Trust (UBHT), which runs the Bristol Royal Infirmary among others in the city, where the real turnaround seems to have occurred.

AFTER a zero rating for the past three years it gained an impressive two stars, making it one of the most improved trusts in the country.

"I am delighted that all the hard work of staff has been rewarded," said trust chief executive, Ron Kerr. "We are one of the few trusts in the country to have made such significant improvement in the space of a year. This is a really good platform on which to build."

Christina Craig, director of performance at the Avon, Gloucestershire and Wiltshire Health Authority, which overlooks the works of all the trusts, welcomed the ratings overall.

"These results are very encouraging for our health community and a credit to the really hard work of the frontline NHS staff," she said. "Some organisations are still not performing at the standard of which we know they are capable and we are supportive of them. They are making significant changes. The result next year will be more positive for them all."

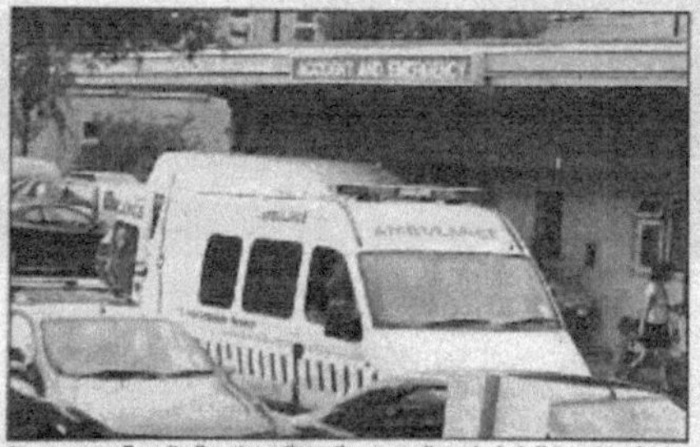

Emergency: Despite the star ratings the commitment of staff is not in doubt

DailyPress How your local NHS fared

ACUTE/ SPECIALIST TRUSTS
- North Bristol NHS Trust: *
- Royal United Hospital Bath NHS Trust: *
- United Bristol Healthcare NHS Trust: **
- Weston Area Health NHS Trust: 0

PRIMARY CARE TRUSTS
- Bath and North East Somerset: **
- Bristol North: **
- Bristol South and West: **
- North Somerset: 0
- South Gloucestershire: **

AMBULANCE TRUSTS
- Avon Ambulance Service NHS Trust: 0

MENTAL HEALTH TRUSTS
- Avon and Wiltshire Mental Health Partnership NHS Trust: **

HCSA articles on whistleblowers in **Hospital Doctor Magazine**

KING POINTS 20 FEBRUARY 2003 • www.hospital-do

NCAA stands by decision not to sacrifice care for speed

Sir, Regarding the article *Poor performers wait 30 weeks for NCAA assessment* (30 January, page 7), the National Clinical Assessment Authority strives to complete assessments as swiftly as possible but this must be consistent with the importance of the concerns we are dealing with.

It is essential that we are addressing the right issues in the right way.

We recognise that for all parties, reaching a resolution quickly is important, which is why we set ourselves a target of 12 weeks. However, we recognised early in our work that there are justifiable reasons why some assessments will take longer.

Our assessments are in-depth and look at all aspects of doctors' performance and the environment in which they work. This takes time, as both doctors and referring bodies need to understand the assessment process and, more importantly, feel comfortable with it.

In addition, many of our assessors and staff at the referring body have commitments which cannot simply be broken, and this can impact on scheduling.

All parties must have sufficient opportunity to engage in the process.

If our recommendations are to work, then both parties need to sign up to them and often the doctor or the referring body quite reasonably request additional time to study these recommendations.

Our referrals continue to rise steadily and we expect continuing growth. We received more referrals in the first six months of this planning year than in the whole of the previous one.

We can assure both doctors and NHS organisations who request our services that we will respond quickly and provide a thorough service, but that we will never sacrifice care to speed.

Dr Alastair Scotland, chief executive and medical director, NCAA

Both clinicians and managers to blame for most suspensions

SUSPENSIONS

THE fault for a doctor's poor performance often lies jointly with the clinical team and trust management, the National Clinical Assessment Authority's (NCAA) annual meeting heard.

In the keynote speech, Prof Sir Liam Donaldson, Chief Medical Officer for England, said only five per cent of consultants felt they had been adequately trained in team leadership skills. Less than half said they had management skills necessary to do the job, compared with 96 per cent who felt they had the clinical skills.

'Often a dysfunctional clinical team is at the heart of the problem,' Sir Liam said.

NCAA chief executive Dr Alastair Scotland said doctors could become personally and professionally isolated even in large hospitals and that such isolation was often a feature of doctors in trouble. 'This shows the importance of clinical governance within teams as well as organisations,' he said.

The NCAA meeting further emphasised the message of team responsibility and support for doctors in difficulty by using actors role-playing as doctors. Delegates, who were mainly chief executives, medical directors, other NHS managers and postgraduate deans, commented on the situations and suggested improvements.

They concluded trusts must have a whistle-blowing policy and that all staff should be aware of it.

They also said a performance advisory panel should deal with concerns raised and its procedures should reflect an 'open, supportive and learning culture'. Trusts should have a named senior officer as an NCAA contact.

Delegates said part of the NCAA's role should be to share good practice with trusts. It should stop using the term 'referral' to describe trusts' informal requests for advice.

A named person within the NCAA should be assigned to handle a problem and the processes should be transparent, they said. Any recommendations should be realistic, timely and consistent.

WEBLINK www.ncaa.nhs.uk

HOW THE NCAA CAN HELP

- **It should share good practice with trusts**
- **It should drop the term 'referral' to describe trusts' informal requests for advice**
- **Recommendations should be realistic, timely and consistent**
- **It should get the funding of recommendations onto the political agenda**

Has your trust improved its record on suspensions, or are doctors still getting a bad deal in your area? Tell us your own experience
E-mail hospital.doctor@rbi.co.uk talkback

12 NEWS 13 NOVEMBER 2003 • www.hospital-doctor.net HOSPITAL DOCTOR

While NCAA was meant to stem suspensions, report questions its operating procedures

Doctors confused by investigators' powers

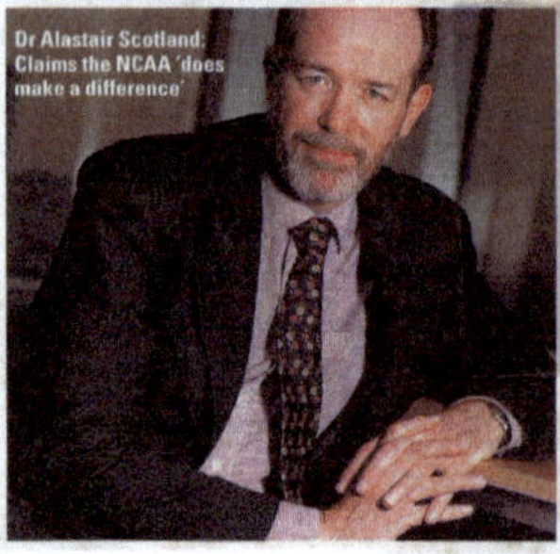

Dr Alastair Scotland: Claims the NCAA 'does make a difference'

by Melanie Newman

SUSPENSIONS

DOCTORS are confused over how the Government's suspension body works.

The National Clinical Assessment Authority (NCAA) was set up by the Government to tackle the number of suspensions in the NHS by providing advice and assistance to trusts and doctors when a problem is identified.

While the National Audit Office (NAO) report says the NCAA has prevented a number of suspensions, some assessed doctors have complained of a lack of clarity about the timetable for the process. Doctors were also uncertain about which doctors were to be interviewed, what cases were to be reviewed and how comments on draft reports were to be incorporated.

Hospital Doctor reported last week that the NAO estimated the costs of suspensions to the NHS at £29m a year.

'Some doctors commented on the critical attitude of the assessment team and its objectivity in weighing evidence,' the report said. It added that almost a third of trusts rated the NCAA's advice as not very or not all effective.

Following publication of the report, the Medical Defence Union called on trusts to make greater use of the NCAA to avoid unnecessary suspensions.

Dr Paul Colbrook, medico-legal adviser at the MDU, said: 'Our experience is that the NCAA's involvement early on can prevent unnecessary suspensions.'

The NCAA's own evaluation report, published in July, said doctors were 'rarely accepting of the need for the assessment', but found assessors supportive and helpful.

A spokeswoman, responding to the NAO report, added: 'Our own evaluation of assessed doctors did not suggest that timing and clarity were foremost in their minds.'

CURE TO SUSPENSION CRISIS LIES WITH TRUST MANAGERS see page

WEBLINK www.nao.gov.uk

HOSPITAL DOCTOR www.hospital-doctor.net • 30 OCTOBER 2003

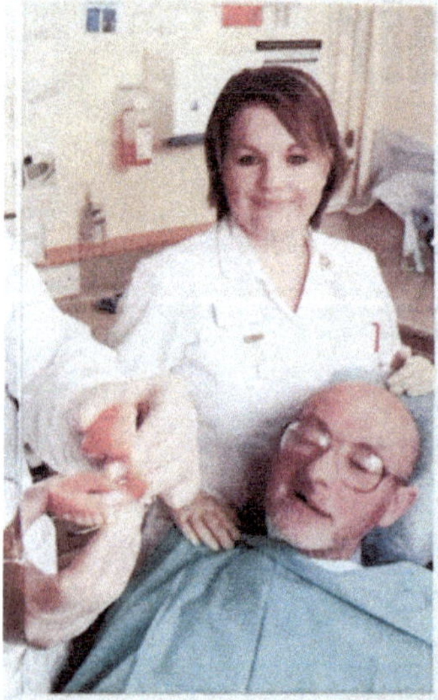

ALL SMILES: Dr Vinod Joshi, a consultant in restorative dentistry at St Luke's Hospital in Bradford, Yorkshire, has led his team in developing a dedicated service for oncological oral care and a website on which patients can share their experiences. He is a finalist in the oncology category of the Hospital Doctor Awards. Full details on page 32

Doctor suspensions 'cost £50m each year'

SUSPENSIONS

THE NHS spends £50m a year on paying suspended doctors to stay at home, hiring replacements and funding investigations into trivial complaints, according to a report.

An article in the *Readers' Digest* said one or two doctors are suspended each week, compared with one or two per month 30 years ago, and that around 100 doctors are currently suspended.

'Most seem to be punishment for whistle-blowing or related to petty jealousies, rows over money and private practice, and arguments with colleagues or managers,' the magazine said. It added that four out of five doctors are cleared after investigations.

The National Audit Office is currently investigating the issue of doctor suspensions. A comprehensive report covering the cost to the health service and the role of the National Clinical Assessment Authority is due in November.

A Private Member's Bill, backed by *Hospital Doctor*, went before the House of Lords in 2000, calling for fairer procedures for doctors.

SEE THE FRONT PAGE FOR MORE ON DISCIPLINARY PROCEDURES

30 OCTOBER 2003 EVERY THURSDAY www.hospital-doctor.net

HOSPITAL

INSIDE THIS WEEK'S *HOSPITAL DOCTOR*

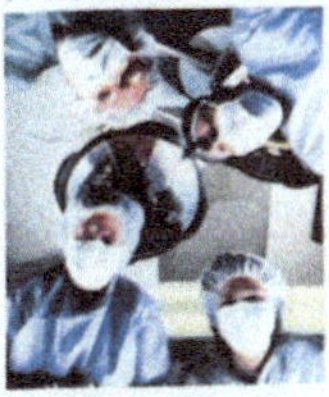

Low SpR vote

With a 37 per cent turnout, what stopped SpRs voting on contract ballot? page 13

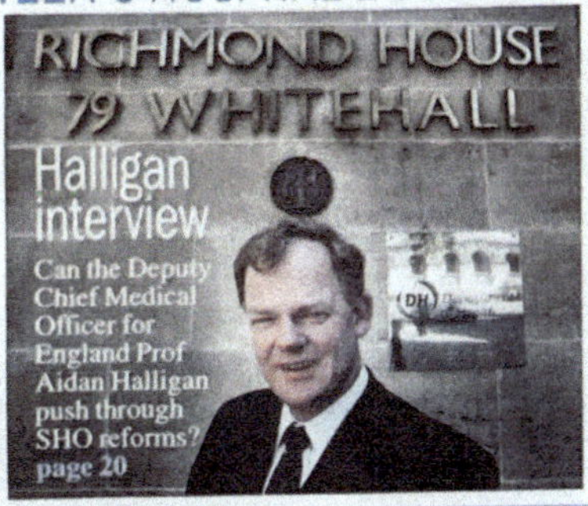

Halligan interview

Can the Deputy Chief Medical Officer for England Prof Aidan Halligan push through SHO reforms? page 20

Suspension propo
accused of unfair

by Melanie Newman

EXCLUSIVE

PROPOSALS for disciplinary and suspension procedures under the new consultant contract have been criticised for failing to allow for fully independent investigations.

A draft document, obtained by *Hospital Doctor*, says concerns about a doctor's practice will be handled by 'appropriately trained individuals locally', but contains no provision for a wholly independent appeals procedure.

Draft framework for discipline and suspension

- **Its remit is clinical performance — local trust procedures will govern conduct issues**
- **Investigations into a doctor's practice to be handled by 'appropriately trained individuals locally'**
- **Trust must notify and seek advice from the National Clinical Assessment Authority**
- **Disciplinary action and 'exclusion' should be last resorts**

The framework — details of which were unavailable during the contract ballot — provides for a 'capability hearing' before trust executive and non-executive directors.

Dr Peter Tomlin, who leads campaigns to make suspension procedures fairer, said: 'There appears to be no proper independent appeal mechanism against reckless and ruthless suspensions by trusts.'

Dr Tomlin, secretary of the Society of Clinical Psychiatrists' study group on suspended doctors, added: 'Any investigation into a doctor's practice should be carried out by people who have no vested interest in local affairs.'

The document discussed by the Department of Health and the BMA says: 'The practitioner will be able to respond to any investigation report, appear before the panel, question any witnesses and be accompanied by a companion.'

But it adds: 'The companion can be legally qualified but will not be acting in a legal capacity.' It is unclear who would be able to request the capability hearing and if 'companions' would be able to cross-examine witnesses.

There would be a right to appeal to a local panel chaired by 'an independent individual from an approved pool'.

'Totally spurious' investigations are crippling our hospitals

Scandal of the NHS doctors paid £50m to stay at home

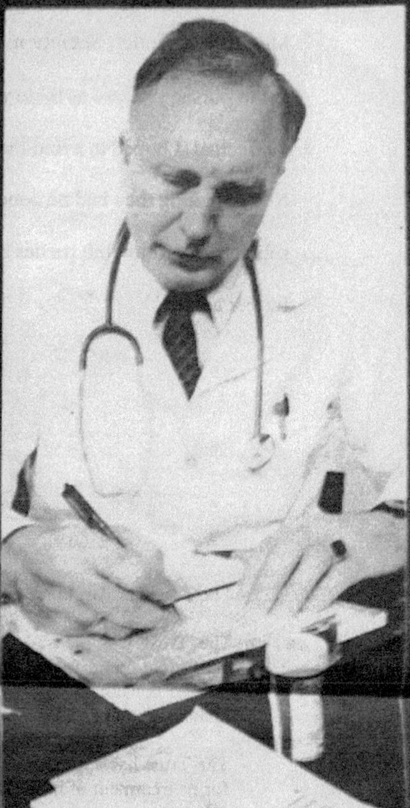

By Ruth Wood

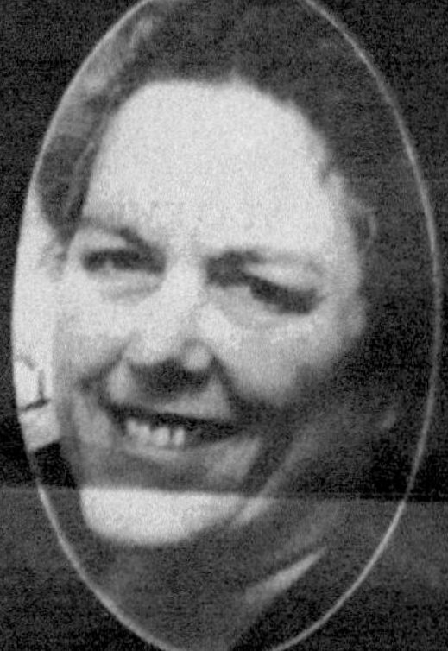

Whistle-blowers being punished

Public Inquiries continued

Bristol heart scandal: In the late 1990s, it was discovered that high mortality rates were occurring in paediatric cardiac surgery at Bristol Royal Infirmary. An inquiry conducted from 1998 to **2001** revealed inadequate care, lack of expertise, and poor communication, resulting in avoidable deaths and complications. (*See below when I met Steve Bolsin at his lecture in Leicester on 14.08.16.)

Harold Shipman: A general practitioner, Harold Shipman, was found to have killed an estimated 215 patients between 1975 and 1998. A public inquiry into his actions was conducted from 2000 to **2002,** which led to significant changes in the system to prevent similar incidents.

Baby P case: This high-profile case involved the death of a 17-month-old boy, known as Baby P, in **2007**. The child suffered severe abuse and neglect despite multiple visits by social workers, doctors, and police. An inquiry examined the failings of the various agencies involved and highlighted the need for better communication and coordination in child protection cases.

Winterbourne View: 2011 Mental health and learning disability care: There have been numerous investigations into the inadequate care and treatment of patients with mental health conditions and learning disabilities. These inquiries have highlighted issues such as inappropriate use of restraint, lack of accessible and quality care, and failures in safeguarding vulnerable individuals.

Liverpool Care Pathway: The Liverpool Care Pathway (LCP), a framework used to manage end-of-life care, came under scrutiny for allegations of inadequate implementation and improper use, with reports of patients being placed on the pathway without appropriate consent. An independent review was conducted in **2013** to assess the concerns and recommend improvements to end-of-life care practices.

Gosport War Memorial Hospital: An investigation was carried out into the practices at Gosport War Memorial Hospital, where it was discovered that the inappropriate prescribing and administering of opioids led to the deaths of hundreds of patients between **1988 and 2000**. A report published in **2018** highlighted the failures in care and management at the facility.

Tainted Blood Scandal: The contaminated blood scandal refers to the use of infected blood products in the NHS during the 1970s and 1980s, which led to thousands of patients contracting HIV and hepatitis C. An inquiry named the Infected Blood Inquiry was established in **2017** to investigate the extent of the failures, subsequent cover-ups, and provide justice for those affected.

Ian Paterson breast surgery scandal: Surgeon Ian Paterson was found guilty in **2017** of performing unnecessary and incorrect breast surgeries on numerous patients. An independent inquiry was launched to examine the circumstances surrounding the case and identify areas where lessons could be learned to prevent similar incidents in the future.

Cervical screening scandal: In **2018**, a national scandal emerged when it was revealed that there were serious errors in the cervical screening programme in England. Many women were not informed about abnormal test results, leading to delayed diagnoses and, in some cases, preventable deaths. An independent review was commissioned to investigate this issue and recommend improvements.

Breast screening programme: 2018. Computer error, no call to final screening of thousands of women aged between 68 to 71 since 2009, totalling 450,000 cases often leading to poorer outcomes. Professor Sir Mike Richards identified the causes of the delays and recommended improvements to the diagnostic processes.

Telford healthcare scandal: In **2018,** an investigation was launched into reports of inappropriate prescribing of medication and poor care at Telford and Wrekin Clinical Commissioning Group. The investigation aimed to determine the extent of the failings and identify areas for improvement.

Whorlton Hall abuse scandal: In **2019**, undercover footage emerged showing staff members at Whorlton Hall, a residential care home for adults with learning disabilities, mistreating and abusing vulnerable patients. The scandal led to multiple investigations and inquiries into the quality of care provided, safeguarding failures, and the effectiveness of regulatory oversight within the UK's health and social care system.

Mesh Scandal inquiry: **2020**, Cumberlege Review investigating the severe complications caused by vaginal mesh implants, leading to significant harm for women.

Letby baby deaths 2023. June 2016, almost a year since Stephen Brearey, the lead doctor at a neonatal unit first became concerned as five babies had died, and at least six others had experienced unusual complications in the neonatal ward at the Countess of Chester Hospital. The number of deaths was far above average for the unit. On June 23, a baby boy — one of a set of newborn triplets — suddenly became sick and died. The following night another of the triplets died. The infants had been in the care of Lucy Letby. Dr Brearey had noticed that she was present in every other suspicious case and raised that fact multiple times with executives, but he felt his concerns were dismissed. After the second triplet died, he phoned a hospital executive and demanded that Ms Letby be removed from the ward. The executive said there was no clear evidence against the nurse and insisted she was safe to work with. It was a week before Ms Letby was moved to clerical duties and months before the hospital's senior managers contacted the police. She was convicted of killing those boys by injecting air into their bodies, murdering five other babies and attempting to murder six others in her care. Since writing this, an appeal has been lodged for a retrial.

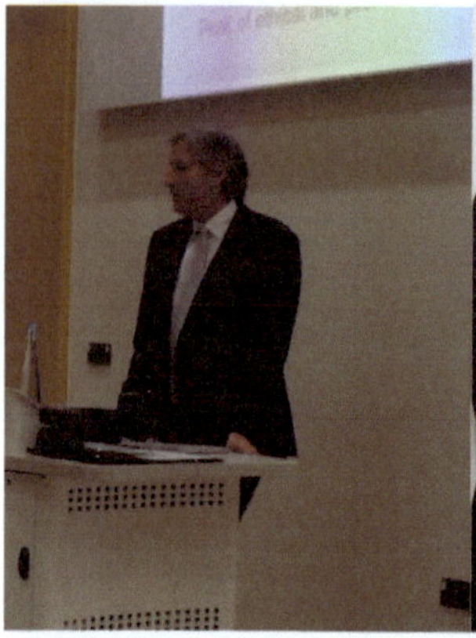

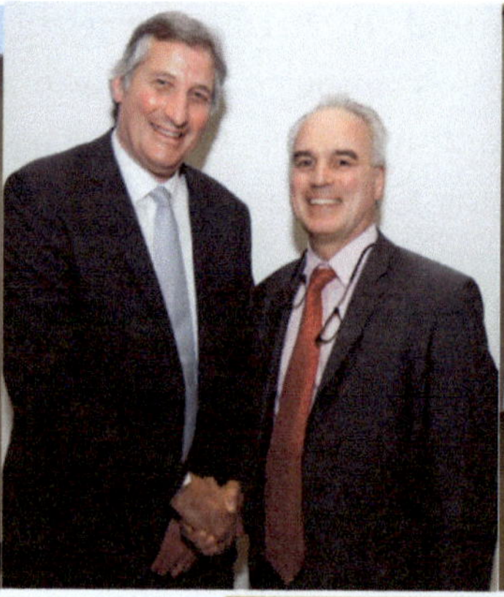

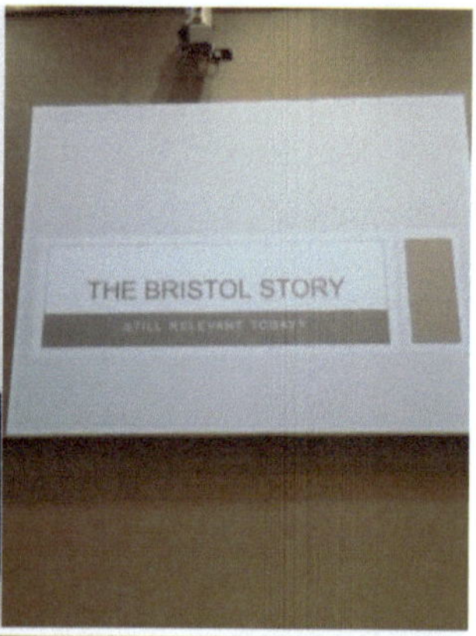
THE BRISTOL STORY
STILL RELEVANT TODAY?

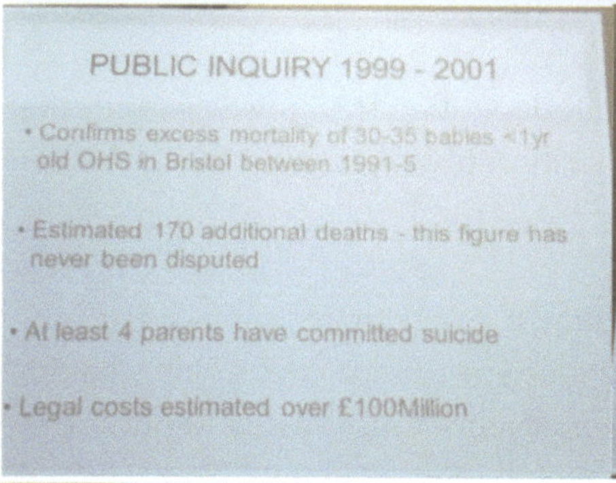
PUBLIC INQUIRY 1999 - 2001
• Confirms excess mortality of 30-35 babies <1yr old OHS in Bristol between 1991-5
• Estimated 170 additional deaths - this figure has never been disputed
• At least 4 parents have committed suicide
• Legal costs estimated over £100Million

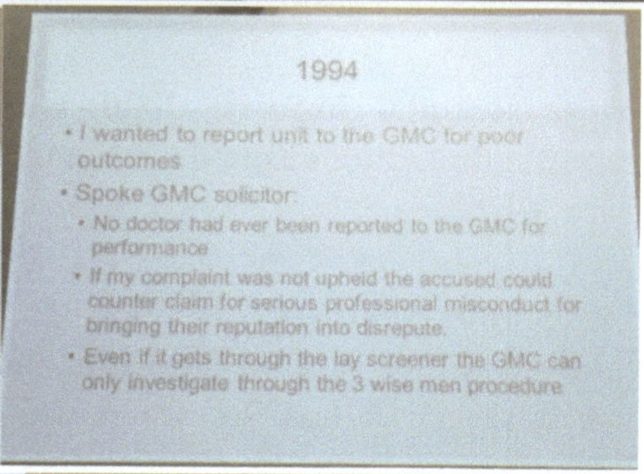
1994
• I wanted to report unit to the GMC for poor outcomes
• Spoke GMC solicitor:
• No doctor had ever been reported to the GMC for performance
• If my complaint was not upheld the accused could counter claim for serious professional misconduct for bringing their reputation into disrepute.
• Even if it gets through the lay screener the GMC can only investigate through the 3 wise men procedure

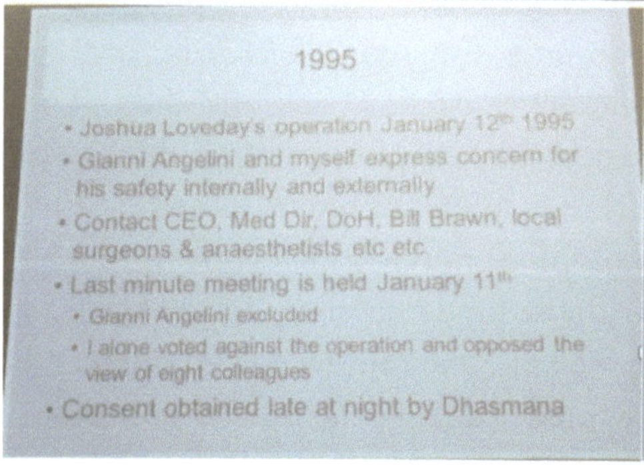
1995
• Joshua Loveday's operation January 12th 1995
• Gianni Angelini and myself express concern for his safety internally and externally
• Contact CEO, Med Dir, DoH, Bill Brawn, local surgeons & anaesthetists etc etc
• Last minute meeting is held January 11th
• Gianni Angelini excluded
• I alone voted against the operation and opposed the view of eight colleagues
• Consent obtained late at night by Dhasmana

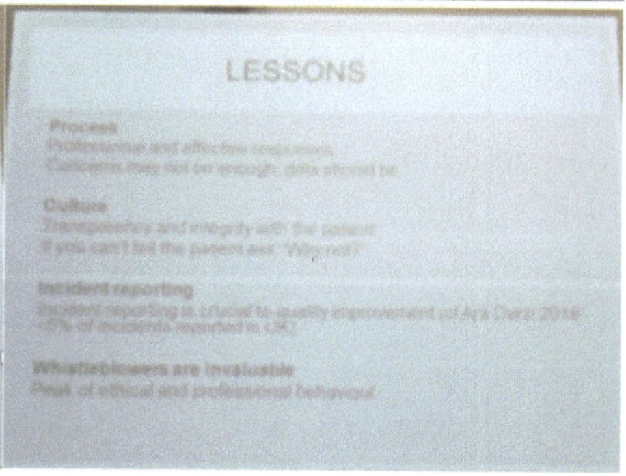
LESSONS
Process
Culture
Incident reporting
Whistleblowers are invaluable
Peak of ethical and professional behaviour

CQC Reports and Locums

Source: https://www.cqc.org.uk

Locum Consultant Cardiologist Yeovil DH NHS Trust 02.05.23 - 06.03.24

20-21 November 2023 the CQC inspection carried out a short-notice announced focused inspection of the maternity service, looking only at the safe and well-led key questions. This was the first time we inspected Yeovil District Hospital maternity services since the merger of two organisations. The rating of this hospital went down. We rated it as requires improvement because the rating of inadequate for maternity services. For the hospital overall it was rated safe as inadequate and well-led as Inadequate. On 8 May 2019 Medical care (including older people's care and Urgent and emergency services rated good and critical care on 27 July 2016 was good.

Subsequently the CQC visited on 13 January to 11 February 2025 to assess the Children and Young People Service due to new and emerging risk. It rated this service as Inadequate. The Yeovil District Hospital is one of 12 NHS Trusts under a national investigation into maternity and neonatal care, led by Baroness Valerie Amos. In May 2025 Yeovil Hospital had taken the decision to close both its Special Care Baby Unit (SCBU) and Maternity Unit for an initial period of six months following safety concerns.

Locum Consultant Acute Physician QEQM Hospital Margate 15.09.21 - 14.10.22

The most recent CQC inspection of QEQM Hospital took place in 2019, and the overall rating given was "Requires Improvement." The CQC found that the hospital provided safe, effective, and caring services, but that there were areas where improvements were needed. The hospital was rated as "Requires Improvement" in the categories of safety, responsiveness, and leadership.

The CQC report highlighted several positive aspects of the care provided by the hospital, including that patients were treated with dignity and respect, that staff were caring and compassionate, and that the hospital had a strong culture of safety and learning. However, the report also identified areas where the hospital could improve, such as reducing the length of time patients wait for treatment, improving the management of medicines, and ensuring that there are enough staff to provide safe and effective care.

Locum Consultant Cardiologist Withy Bush and Glangwili Carmargen Hospitals 08.12.20 - 11.05.21

Healthcare Inspectorate Wales (HIW). The latest HIW inspection of Withybush General Hospital took place in 2019, and the overall rating given was "Adequate." to improve, such as ensuring that there were enough staff with the right skills to provide safe and effective care, improving the management of patient records, and addressing issues with the cleanliness and maintenance of the hospital.

Locum Consultant Cardiologist Colchester Hospital University Foundation Trust 21.09.20 - 04.12.20

The most recent CQC inspection of Colchester Hospital took place in 2019, and the overall rating given was "Requires Improvement." The CQC found that the hospital provided safe, effective, and caring services, but that there were areas where improvements were needed. The hospital was rated as "Requires Improvement" in the categories of safety, responsiveness, and well-led.

Locum Consultant Cardiologist North Cumbria NHS Acute Hospitals NHS Trust 10.08.20 - 18.09.20

The most recent CQC inspection of North Cumbria Integrated Care NHS Foundation Trust took place in 2019, and the overall rating given was "Requires Improvement." The CQC found that the Trust provided safe, effective, and caring services, but there were areas where improvements were needed. The Trust was rated as "Requires Improvement" in the categories of responsiveness and leadership.

Locum Consultant Cardiologist West Suffolk Hospital NHS Trust 30.03.20 - 17.07.20

The most recent CQC inspection of West Suffolk Hospital took place in 2018, and the overall rating given was "Good." The CQC found that the hospital provided safe, effective, caring, responsive, and well-led services. The hospital was rated as "Good" in all categories.

Locum Consultant Cardiologist Conquest Hospital NHS Trust Hastings 11.02.20 - 06.03.20

The most recent CQC inspection of Conquest Hospital took place in 2019, and the overall rating given was "Requires Improvement." The CQC found that the hospital provided safe, effective, and caring services, but that there were areas where improvements were needed.

The hospital was rated as "Requires Improvement" in the categories of responsiveness and leadership.

Locum Cardiologist QEQM Hospital, East Kent University NHS Foundation Trust 20.01.20 - 31.01.20

The most recent CQC inspection of QEQM Hospital took place in 2019, and the overall rating given was "Requires Improvement." The CQC found that the hospital provided safe, effective, and caring services, but that there were areas where improvements were needed. The hospital was rated as "Requires Improvement" in the categories of safety, responsiveness, and leadership.

The CQC report highlighted several positive aspects of the care provided by the hospital, including that patients were treated with dignity and respect, that staff were caring and compassionate, and that the hospital had a strong culture of safety and learning. However, the report also identified areas where the hospital could improve, such as reducing the length of time patients wait for treatment, improving the management of medicines, and ensuring that there are enough staff to provide safe and effective care.

Locum Cardiologist Doncaster Royal and Bassetlaw NHS Trust 02.12.19 - 23.12.19

The most recent CQC inspection of Doncaster and Bassetlaw Teaching Hospitals NHS Foundation Trust took place in 2019, and the overall rating given was "Requires Improvement." The CQC found that the trust provided safe, effective, and caring services, but that there were areas where improvements were needed. The trust was rated as "Requires Improvement" in the categories of responsiveness and leadership.

Locum Cardiologist Wolverhampton NHS Trust 30.09.19 - 29.11.19

The most recent CQC inspection of Wolverhampton NHS Trust took place in 2019, and the overall rating given was "Requires Improvement." The CQC found that the trust provided safe, effective, and caring services, but that there were areas where improvements were needed. The trust was rated as "Requires Improvement" in the categories of responsiveness and leadership.

Locum Cardiologist Salisbury District Hospital 13.08.19 - 13.09.19

The most recent CQC inspection of the Salisbury NHS Foundation Trust took place in 2019, and the overall rating given was "Good." The CQC found that the trust provided safe, effective, caring, responsive, and well-led services. The trust was rated as "Good" in all five categories assessed by the CQC.

Locum Consultant Cardiologist Northampton General Hospital 24.06.19 - 09.08.19

11 June to 25 July 2019

During a routine inspection

Rating of services went down in these areas: 'safe and well-led' required improvement and effective, caring, and responsive as good. Two of the hospital's eight core services require improvement and six as good. They took into account the current ratings of the five services not inspected this time dating from 2017. Mandatory training in key skills was not given to all staff but all did complete it. The trust did not always have enough staff with the right qualifications, skills, training and experience to keep patients safe from avoidable harm and to provide the right care and treatment. Records were not always easily available to all staff providing care. Trust staff did not always follow its systems and processes to safely administer, record and store medicines. Managers did not consistently share lessons learned with the whole team and the wider service and did not always ensure that actions from patient safety alerts were implemented and monitored. People could not always access services when they needed them and as a result did not always receive the right care promptly.

Waiting times from referral to treatment and arrangements to admit, treat and discharge patients were consistently worse than national standards and trust did not achieve NHS constitutional standards in its urgent care service. Complaints were not always managed in line with the trust's own timescales. Staff did not all feel respected, supported and valued, staff feedback and experience showed a culture of bullying behaviour. Not all staff felt that they were kept fully informed or had their views listened to and acted upon and quality measures were not consistently collected in the maternity service.

Locum Consultant Cardiologist and Physician 11.02.19 - 05.04.19
North Devon Hospital Barnstable

The most recent CQC inspection of the Northern Devon Healthcare NHS Trust took place in 2018, and the overall rating given was "Good. The areas where the trust could improve, such as reducing the length of time patients wait for treatment and improving the management of medicines.

Locum Consultant Cardiologist and Physician 29.05.18 - 31.12.18
Warwick Hospital SWFT

The most recent CQC inspection of South Warwickshire NHS Foundation in 2019 found it provided good quality care and made improvements since its last inspection.

Locum Consultant Cardiologist
Arrowe Park Hospital NHS Trust Liverpool 27.11.17 - 18.01.18

The most recent CQC inspection of Arrowe Park Hospital NHS Trust took place in 2018, and the overall rating given was "Good." The CQC found that the trust provided safe, effective, caring, responsive, and well-led services. The trust was rated as "Good" in all five categories assessed by the CQC. It made improvements since its last inspection. The trust has since been working to make further improvements

Locum Consultant Cardiologist 30.08.17 - 03.11.17
and Physician Yeovil District Hospital NHS Trust
The most recent CQC inspection of Yeovil District Hospital NHS Trust took place in 2019, and the overall rating given was "Requires Improvement." The CQC identified some areas where improvements were needed, including in the management of medicines, the responsiveness of services to patients' needs, and the effectiveness of leadership. The trust was also rated as "Requires Improvement" in the "Safe" and "Well-led" categories.

Locum Consultant Cardiologist 31.10.16 - 05.05.17
Homerton University Hospital NHS Trust
The most recent CQC inspection of Homerton University Hospital NHS Trust took place in 2011 and overall rating was good." The CQC found it provided safe, effective, caring responsive and well-led services. Improved since last inspection, rated 'Good' in all 5 categories.

Honorary Cardiologist University of July 2011 - Nov 2016
Coventry and Warwickshire NHS Trust
Dr Mattu said he had been 'vilified and bullied' after making claims about care at the Walsgrave Hospital in Coventry in 2001. University Hospitals Coventry and Warwickshire submitted over 200 false allegations about him to the General Medical Council, resulting in the cardiologist being investigated from 2002 to 2009 and 2011 to 2013, the UK's most investigated doctor by the GMC. Commission for Health Improvement gave the hospital a 'zero star rating' in 2001,

Locum Consultant West Hertfordshire NHS
Trust Watford General Hospital Sept' 2016 - Oct' 2016
The most recent CQC inspection of West Hertfordshire NHS Trust took place in 2019, and the overall rating given was "Requires Improvement." The CQC identified some areas where improvements were needed, including in the management

of medicines, the responsiveness of services to patients' needs, and the effectiveness of leadership.

The trust was also rated as "Requires Improvement" in the "Safe" and "Well-led" categories, while it was rated as "Good" in the "Caring" category.

Locum Consultant Gloucester Royal Hospital July 2015 - Aug' 2015

0-13 March 2015, and 20 March 2015 During a routine inspection overall, Gloucestershire Royal Hospital was rated as requiring improvement. We rated it as good for caring and as requiring improvements in safety, effectiveness, being responsive to patients' needs and being well led. Overall, critical care was rated as outstanding. Urgent and emergency care and medicine required improvement; all other services were rated as good. Maternity and gynaecology and services for children and young people were rated as good with the remaining core services rated as requiring improvement.

Locum Consultant Cardiologist Douglas Isle of Man March 2015 -June 2015

The West Midlands Quality Review Service found more than 50% of areas within the island's critical care department to be underperforming. The first phase of the £200,000 review looked into Accident and Emergency, Theatres and Anaesthetics and Critical care. Health Minister Howard Quayle said the review inspectors expressed concern about a "culture of blame" within the hospital.

Locum Consultant Medway Hospital, Gillingham Dec' 2014 - Feb' 2015

On 31 December 2013 we carried out an unannounced inspection of the Emergency Department (ED) at Medway Maritime Hospital in response to information received from an anonymous source regarding the safety and effectiveness of the ED. CQC found that the service was failing to meet the national standards that people should expect to receive. As a result, issued formal warning notices to Medway NHS Foundation Trust, telling them that they must improve in a number of areas within a specified period of time. Further unannounced inspections of the ED on 27 and 28 July 2014 and again on 26 August 2014. On 28 July 2014 also reviewed the surgery department to determine whether the trust had made the necessary improvements to the service and inspections of the ED in July and August 2014, found ED lacked robust clinical leadership.

Locum Consultant Pilgrim Hospital Boston October 2014

A routine inspection of the Pilgrim Hospital was made on 1 and 2 May 2014 as part of the wider inspection of United Lincolnshire Hospitals NHS Trust. The trust was chosen for inspection because it was an example of a 'high risk' trust. Sir Bruce Keogh's review (Keogh Mortality Review) in 2013 found significant concerns and the trust was placed in 'special measures' as a result.

The hospital was rated as requiring improvement. Core services for accident and emergency (A&E), medical care, surgery and maternity were found, overall, to require improvement.

The previous year it was inspected on 21, 25 June and 2, 4, 5 July 2013 when the Care Quality Commission was contacted by the Bruce Keogh Rapid Response Team, as they had concerns about the staffing levels at the hospital, particularly at night and weekends. The CQC undertook three unannounced inspections to the hospital, one on a Friday night. Staff were not confident in the reporting system and told us that feedback was inconsistent between managers. One doctor said, 'I don't think anything is being fed up to the Board, we occasionally and perhaps get an email from the medical directorate about an incident telling us not to do something.'

Locum Consultant Princess Royal Hospital Farnborough Kings College NHS Trust April 2014 – Oct 2014

Prior to being dissolved, the South London Healthcare Trust experienced severe financial challenges, which impacted on many areas of care and systems for monitoring the quality of care provided. The due diligence reports carried out by King's College Hospital NHS Foundation Trust, dated June 2013, identified a number of significant problems, including the processes for managing risk, complaints and clinical effectiveness, which were perceived to be weak and understaffed. Some staff working in clinical areas appeared to have become resigned to the situation and worked around the problems rather than addressing them. This attitude was evident in some interviews with staff and during our observations of clinical areas. The plans of senior managers had not yet had enough visible impact on the delivery of care.

Consultant Cardiologist Barnsley Hospital NHS Trust Feb' 2014 - April 2014
2013 Met CQC standards

Locum Consultant Cardiologist Tameside Hospital NHS Trust Dec' 2013 - Feb' 2014
In 2013, the trust was identified nationally as having high mortality rates and it was one of 14 hospital trusts to be investigated by Sir Bruce Keogh (the Medical Director for NHS England) as part of the Keogh Mortality Review in July that year. After that review, the trust entered special measures because there were concerns about the care of emergency patients and those whose conditions might deteriorate. There were also concerns about staffing levels (particularly of senior medical staff at night and weekends), patients' experiences of care and, more generally, that the Trust Board was too reliant on reassurance rather than explicit assurance about levels of care and safety.

Locum Consultant Cardiologist Ealing Hospital NHS Trust Oct' 2008 - Jan' 2013
Met CQC standards

Locum Consultant Cardiologist Dumfries & Galloway Royal Infirmary Dec' 2007 - April 2008
Healthcare Improvement Scotland previously inspected Dumfries & Galloway Royal Infirmary in January 2014. That inspection resulted in eight requirements and three recommendations. e.g. ensure that all mattresses in use are clean and fit for purpose. This will minimise the risk of cross-contamination from these items of equipment to patients.

Locum Consultant Cardiologist Vale of Leven & Western Infirmary, North Glasgow University Oct' 2004 - Dec' 2007
In the period 1 January 2007 to 31 December 2008 total deaths identified by the Inquiry in which CDI was a causal factor was 34. These figures are in the context of the VOLH, a hospital with around 136 beds in 2008.

Locum Consultant Cardiologist University Hospitals April 2003 - Oct' 2004
Coventry and Warwickshire NHS Trust

Dr Mattu said he had been 'vilified and bullied' after making claims about care at the Walsgrave Hospital in Coventry in 2001. University Hospitals Coventry and Warwickshire submitted over 200 false allegations about him to the General Medical Council, resulting in the cardiologist being investigated from 2002 to 2009 and 2011 to 2013, the UK's most investigated doctor by the GMC. Commission for Health Improvement gave the hospital a 'zero star rating' in 2001

Locum Cons. (Card/Med) Tameside and Glossop NHS Trust Feb' 2003 - April 2003

In 2013, the trust was identified nationally as having high mortality rates and it was one of 14 hospital trusts to be investigated by Sir Bruce Keogh (the Medical Director for NHS England) as part of the Keogh Mortality Review in July that year. After that review, the trust entered special measures because there were concerns about the care of emergency patients and those whose conditions might deteriorate. There were also concerns about staffing levels (particularly of senior medical staff at night and weekends), patients' experiences of care and, more generally, that the Trust Board was too reliant on reassurance rather than explicit assurance about levels of care and safety.

Consultant (Card/Med) Weston General Hospital & Honorary Consultant Cardiologist Jan' 2002 - Dec' 2002
U.B.H.T

(CQC) have inspected Weston General Hospital and published their findings. We last inspected medical care at Weston General Hospital in June 2021 and rated the core service inadequate. In the 2005/2006 period, *On the quality of the healthcare it provided, the hospital was rated as weak on a four-point scale of weak, fair, good and excellent. This placed the hospital in the bottom performing 9% of trusts in the country. On the same scale, the hospital's use of resources was also rated weak, placing it in the bottom 37% of trusts in the country. On 7 July 2003, BBC Television programme Inside Out broadcast allegations from a whistleblower that senior management within the hospital were putting pressure on employees to manipulate waiting list statistics to make them look more favourable. An independent enquiry in 2004 concluded that this manipulation did take place.*

Consultant (Card/Med) West Cumberland Hospital & Honorary Consultant Cardiologist South Cleveland April '95 -Jan' 2002

No CQC reports are available during this period; 18 April 2011

During a themed inspection looking at Dignity and Nutrition Patients we spoke to were mostly very positive about their experience of care and treatment. Most patients said they had their care needs met and had been treated respectfully. A typical comment received was 'There has been no waiting for care, treatment generally has been very good and staff are very caring.' A relative said 'We have been very happy with care in this hospital, we have experienced two hospitals out of the area and this is by far the best for care, and staff treating you right'.

Locum Cons. (Card/Med) Good Hope NHS Trust Feb' 1994-April 1995

No CQC reports are available during this period.

Good Hope Hospital was previously managed by Heart of England NHS Foundation Trust. On 1 April 2018 a merger by acquisition took place of Heart of England NHS Foundation Trust by University Hospitals of Birmingham NHS Foundation Trust. As such Good Hope Hospital is now part of University Hospitals of Birmingham NHS Foundation Trust.

Locum Cons. (Card/Med) Taunton & Somerset Trust Sept' 1993-Feb' 1994

No CQC reports are available during this period.

Musgrove Park Hospital is the largest general hospital in Somerset and is part of the Taunton and Somerset NHS Foundation Trust.

Locum Cons. (Cardiol) Royal Cornwall Hospitals, Truro June 1993-Sept' 1993

No CQC reports are available during this period.

CQC has previously carried out two comprehensive inspections at Royal Cornwall Hospital NHS Trust. The first being in January 2014 when the Trust was rated as requiring improvement.

Acknowledgements

Mentors in training:
David de Bono (Deceased)
Doug Skehan

Supporting colleagues:
John McCrea (Deceased)
Carl Thomson
Tahir Qaseem
Colin Dyan
Peter Glennon
Hardial Singh
ManFei Shu
Martin Been
Robin Roberts
Jaspal Kooner
Stuart Rosen
Madhusudhan Varma
Tim Bowker
Arvinder Kurbaan
Clive Weston
Andrew Broadley
Jonathan Sahu
Sundeep Puree
Jonathan Byrne
Professor Theresa McDonagh
Hugh Carmichael
Douglas McCruden

Others:
BCS Guy Lloyd
John Camm
Sir Bruce Keogh
Sir George Alberti
Sir Robert Francis

Cardiac technicians West Cumberland
All Nursing and technical staff who believed in me
Whistleblowers All published and unknown
PCAW report May 2013

HCSA
Joe Chattin (retired)
Sasha Burn A special thank you to Sasha for her input in relation to employment issues and for reading and advising on so many drafts of the manuscript until the end!

References

1. https://www.bristol-inquiry.org.uk/final_report/the_report.pdf
2. Claire Hilton. Essay; Whistle-blowing and duty of candour in the National Health Service: a 'history and policy' case study of the 1960s and 2010s. *Journal of the Royal Society of Medicine*. 2016, vol 109(9) 327-330.
3. Barnes Gharsgozloo I F, Poston R. Rainer WG Gruessner. Editorial. Consequences for Whistleblowing: Retaliation, Sham Peer Review and Hospital Immunity. *Journal of Biomedical Research & Environmental Sciences*. 2023 Feb 16; 4(2): 235-238.
4. Kingston M, Evans S, Smith B, Berry J. Attitudes of doctors and nurses towards incident reporting: a qualitative analysis *Medical Journal of Australia*. 181: 1, 36-39.
5. Whistleblowing: The Inside Story. A study of the experiences of 1,000 whistleblowers. A research project by Public Concern at Work and the University of Greenwich. May 2013.
6. Dasguota S, Keshharwani A. Whistleblowing: A survey of the literature *The IUP Journal of Corporate Governance*. Vol. IX, No. 4, 2010
7. Jackson D. Peters K, Hutchinson M, et al. Exploring confidentiality in the context of nurse whistle blowing: issues for nurse managers. *Journal of Nursing Management*. vol. 19, no. 5, pp. 655-663.
8. GR, **Forbat LN.** Cervical and Vestibular Afferent Control of Oculomotor Response in Man. *Acta Otolaringol*. 1979; 88:78-87.
9. **Forbat LN**, Brown OC, Shenouda FS. The relationships between Maternal HbA1, Maternal Size and Foetoplacental Size in Indian Pregnancies. *Early Human Development*. 1981; 5: 253-65.
10. **Forbat LN**, Collins RE, Maskell GK, Sonksen PH. Glucose Concentrations in Parotid Fluid and Venous Blood of Patients Attending a Diabetic Clinic. *Journal of the Royal Society of Medicine*. 1981; 74:725-8.
11. Report of the Mid Staffordshire NHS Foundation Trust Public Inquiry: executive summary HC 947, Session 2012-2013 - 0947.pdf
12. Sir Robert Francis. http://freedomtospeakup.org.uk/the-report/

13. The Report of the Morecambe Bay Investigation March 2015 Dr Bill Kirkup CBEhttps://assets.publishing.service.gov.uk/media/5a7f3d7240f0b6230 5b85efb/47487_MBI_Accessible_v0.1.pdf
14. *Queen Elizabeth Queen Mary hospital CQC report* https://www.cqc.org.uk/location/RVV09/inspection-summary
15. Raj Mattu audit trail http://drphilhammond.com/blog/2014/04/25/private-eye/raj-mattu-audit-trail/
16. http://54000doctors.org/thecase/1-intro-and-how-this-case-affects-you.html https://www.bma.org.uk/advice-and-support/nhs-delivery-and-workforce/workforce/consultant-workforce-shortages
17. https://www.rcp.ac.uk/media/qglpgsyq/guidance-for-approving-nhs-specialist-dr-posts-1.pdf
18. Peters K, Luck L, Hutchinson M, Lesley Wilkes, et al. The emotional sequelae of whistleblowing: findings from a qualitative study. *Journal of Clinical Nursing.* 20, 2907–2914.
19. Doctors who commit suicide while under GMC fitness to practise investigation Sandrah Horsfall, Independent Consultant. December 14 2014. https://www.gmc-uk.org/-/media/documents/internal-review-into-suicide-in-ftp-processes_pdf-59088696.pdf
20. Horsfall%202014%20Internal-review-into-suicide-in-FTP-processes_pdf-59088696.pdf
21. https://www.gmc-uk.org/-/media/documents/Internal_review_intosuicide_in-FTP_processes.pdf_59088696.pdf
22. *Dyer C. GMC and vulnerable doctors: too blunt an instrument? BMJ2013; 347:f623*96653493.pdf
23. Leymann H (2004) Bullying; Whistleblowing, the Discovery of PTSD as a Diagnosis Victimisation at Work. The Mobbing Encyclopaedia. Available at: http://www.leymann.se/English/frame. html (accessed 28 October 2004)
24. https://wessex.hee.nhs.uk/wp-content/uploads/sites/6/2020/04/keogh-review-final-report.pdf
25. nhs-digital-foi-disclosure-15.02.2019-ref-nic-264888-t2d3x-reason-for-leaving-dismissal-some-other-substantial-reason_ (archived)
26. 'Dysfunctional' GMC Labelled 'Not Fit for Purpose' After Latest Blunder. Dr Sheena Meredith, MB BS, MPhil. November 10 2022 https://www.medscape.co.uk/viewarticle/dysfunctional-gmc-labelled-not-fit-purpose-after-latest-2022a100260x
27. Compendium-of-GMC-published-findings-relating-to-Fitness-to-Practise-rates_pdf

28. https://www.gmc-uk.org/news/news-archive/co-chairs-of-dr-arora-case-review-publish-findings
29. Clare Dyer. Whistleblower was unfairly dismissed in case lasting 12 years, tribunal rules *The BMJ*. 2014; 348
30. Christie B. Lack of leadership was at the heart of hospital's failings, report says. *The BMJ*. 2015;351:n3799doi:10.1136/bmj.h3799 pmid:26162915
31. Christie B. Troubled Aberdeen hospital is back in spotlight. *The BMJ*. 201; 350:h3254. Doi:10.1136/bmj.h3354 pmid:26070478
32. Christie B. "Unacceptable behaviour" may lead to action against senior doctors at Aberdeen hospital. *The BMJ*. 2014;349:g7483. Doi:10.1136/bmj.g7483 pmid:25477527.
33. Justin Waring. When Whistle-blowers Become the Story: The Problem of the 'Third Victim'; Comment on "Cultures of Silence and Cultures of Voice: The Role of Whistleblowing in Healthcare Organisations" *International Journal of Health Policy Management*. 2016, 5(2), 133-135
34. Christie B. GMC closes inquiry into troubled Aberdeen hospital BMJ 27 September 2016;354:i15250 doi: 10.1136/bmj.i5250
35. Bewick Report: Professor Mike Bewick, Independent Health Consultant and founder iQ4U Consultants Ltd. Dr Simon Haynes, Consultant Paediatric Cardiac Anaesthetist, Newcastle Hospital Foundation Trust. Period of Review 11th June to 3rd July. https://www.stgeorges.nhs.uk/wp-content/uploads/2018/08/Independent-review-of-cardiac-surgery-%E2%80%93-St-George%E2%80%99s-University-Hospitals....pdf
36. David Nichol. Whistleblowing: what progress since the Francis Inquiry report? BMJ 2019;364:l1482
37. https://www.gov.uk/government/publications/report-of-the-mid-staffordshire-nhs-foundation-trust-public-inquiry
38. Berman A. Ogden G. Whistleblowing in the NHS – freedom to speak up: a summary. Dental Update, 44(6), 571-574
39. Bolsin S, Faunce T, Oakley J. Practical virtue ethics: healthcare whistleblowing and portable digital technology. *Journal of Medical Ethics*. 2005; 31:612–618.
40. Word (2003) Whistleblowing: When It Works and Why, *Public Integrity*. 5:4, 373-375. Solutions
41. Jackson D, Peters K, Andrew S. et al. Understanding whistleblowing: Qualitative insights from nurse whistleblowers. October 2010. *Journal of Advanced Nursing* 66(10):2194-201.
42. Mannion R, Blenkinsopp J, Powell M, et al. Understanding the knowledge gaps in whistleblowing and speaking up in health care: narrative reviews of

the research literature and formal inquiries, a legal analysis and stakeholder interviews. *Health and Social Care Delivery Research.* 2018;6(30):1–190.

43. Dr. Purnima Sehgal. Can Whistleblowers live Happily Ever After? A Review of Literature on Whistleblowing and its Implications. *IRJMST* Vol 8 Issue 1 [Year 2017] ISSN 2250 – 1959
44. Aoed Jone. The Role of Employee Whistleblowing and Raising Concerns in an Organisational Learning Culture – Elusive and Laudable?; Comment on "Cultures of Silence and Cultures of Voice: The Role of Whistleblowing in Healthcare Organisations", *International Journal of Health Policy Management.* 2016, 5(1), 67–69
45. D. Robert MacDougall. Whistleblowing: Don't Encourage It, Prevent It; Comment on "Cultures of Silence And Cultures of Voice: The Role Of Whistleblowing in Healthcare Organisations". *International Journal of Health Policy Management.* 2016, 5(3), 189–191
46. Mannion R, Davies H. Cultures of Silence and Cultures of Voice: The Role of Whistleblowing in Healthcare Organisation. *International Journal of Health Policy Management.* 2015, 4(8), 503–505
47. T Faunce, S Bolsin, W-P Chan. THE OLIVIERI SYMPOSIUM Supporting whistleblowers in academic medicine: training and respecting the courage of professional conscience. *Journal of Medical Ethics.* 2004; 30:40–43
48. Peter B. Jubb. Whistleblowing: A Restrictive. Definition and Interpretation *Journal of Business Ethics.* 21: 77–94, 1999.
49. Charles Frederick Alford. What Makes Whistleblowers So Threatening?; Comment on "Cultures of Silence and Cultures of Voice: The Role of Whistleblowing in Healthcare Organisations". *International Journal of Health Policy Management.* 2016, 5(1), 71–73
50. Rhodes R. Strain J. Whistleblowing in academic medicine. *Journal of Medical Ethics.* 2004;30:35–39
51. Lewis & Vandekerckhove. The Content of Whistleblowing Procedures: A Critical review of Recent Official guidelines. *Journal of Business Ethics.* (2011) 1-30.
52. https://www.england.nhs.uk/long-read/retaining-doctors-in-late-stage-career/https://hansard.parliament.uk/commons/20020117/debates/42aa7a61-6e52-48c8-bccc-fa78aad535b6/BristolRoyalInfirmary#contribution-502c783d-4161-43e0-866c-da943469b84d
53. Taylor D. Goodwin D. Organisational failure: rethinking whistleblowing for tomorrow's doctors. *Journal of Medical Ethics.* 2022; 48:672–677
54. Health and Social Care Act 2008 (Regulated activities) Regulations 2014. Regulation 20
55. https://www.gmc-uk.org/about/what-we-do-and-why/our-mandate

Interview with Nick Ferrari on LBC 17.05.24

My transcript is from the original recording on LBC catch-up

"Nick Ferrari
The most comprehensive NHS review – they point to teetering Social care system harder for staff to free up beds and we growing older and in many instances, growing sicker, if that's the correct fashion, as we require more care also throw in the fact that strikes of course have blighted parts of the health service and it's a pretty toxic mix isn't it, so does that speak to you? Are you safely at home now but you had trouble getting out does it speech as I said earlier, an elderly relative or loved one and you are, because we are more mobile you want a different part of the country you're not able to provide the care you on and it has been a nightmare trying to sort getting dad out of a hospital or granddad or whatever. How big a deal is this, well **let's bring Doctor Tim Cooksley who's immediate past president of The Society for Acute Medicine** into the conversation and it looks very grim from these headlines doctor, but you've been at the coalface as it were what the reality is you see it? Good morning.

Tim Cooksley
Good morning, Nick. I think unfortunately outlined it perfectly there as you know we have had for the last couple of years consistently over 10,000 older frailer patients in hospital every day who would be better looked after that own homes supported by community services and not just led to hopefully can be overcrowded, real problems in our emergency departments and acute medical services, and also a long waiting list as we haven't got enough space to get people in for procedures and surgery, so this is an ongoing serious problem that of course is exacer*bated by the fact*

learning people get poorly in their own home and could traditionally have been looked after by 'at home' and community services. They aren't there so they end up in corridors in acute *medical units and emergency departments,* and all these awful experiences people are having.

Nick Ferrari
So, doctor, what is worsening the picture as it were, is it, unfortunately, we have even less and less cash going into social care? Is it a social care system that effectively doesn't exist? Is it because people down to the brilliance of people like you and your colleagues, you are keeping people alive longer who wouldn't have been around to cause issues years ago?

Tim Cooksley
It's a combination of all these things, they can of course we've known for a long time that people are going to get older and live longer with more complex conditions and we haven't planned for that this isn't a surprise and this will continue to happen and we need to have a sustainable long term plan actually works out how we're going to look after people with these complex illnesses *and getting older and that's expensive* and it needs staff and it needs increased community services and there's some short term things we can do, but it means that long term plan that we're not having this conversation again in 10 years' time.

Nick Ferrari
Well, amen to that. It can only be down to the brilliance of your colleagues if I am still here in 10 years' time, but what are the main pillars that need to be imposed put in place then for that reform, would you say doctor?

Tim Cooksley
So in terms of helping people to get out of hospital it's going to be community services with increased district nurses, GPs and care within the community, helping look after these patients. I will see a number *patients* today on my *ward round* on the acute medical unit who don't need to be in hospital per se but do need care, complex nursing services and support from expert GP

colleagues in the community. And those are the services which we haven't funded satisfactorily, *alongside all the other things that are happening inside our emergency department and acute medical units.*

Nick Ferrari
Lastly, does there need to be more joined-up thinking in the sense between different branches of the NHS and different branches of local authority care?

Tim Cooksley
Absolutely there does and of course when people are so strained, this is where things fall down. We need capacity throughout the system so that colleagues can work optimally, provide high-quality care so that we communicate carefully, so that communication is there, so people don't fall through the cracks.

Nick Ferrari
I'll let you get off to the fantastic work your colleagues do. Thanks to you, Dr Tim Cooksley, immediate past president of The Society of Acute Medicine. He will be on his rounds I imagine within minutes or certainly later this morning. Lance, coming to you as the first caller in just a moment as you have a key voice in this, but it's worth remembering former chancellor, we're talking about the current one later. Sir Nigel Lawson once said the NHS is the closest thing the English have to a religion, I am sure if you reviewed his words he would say the British, I am sure he would. It is the closest thing we have to a faith effectively now for many people in this country, but we have to, we have to be honest critics and arbiters of it. Clearly this isn't working, there have probably been, the NHS seems to have a reform as often as Harry Kane changes his socks, but nothing seems to make it better. Why? And this issue now, particularly, I hate that expression, I know it sums it up, 'bed blockers'. But if that is referring to your grandad, it's not particularly polite, is it? He doesn't want to be one. What a ghastly... It's like that. Why did they use to call it joy riding? Do you remember that? Joy riding, nicking a car driving and sometimes crashing it and burning

it. Well, I'm, anyway its call taking and driving away now! **Anyway, let's come back to health Lance is in Bristol, what do you do for a living?** Good morning.

Lance Forbat

Good morning. Thank you Nick, I am a cardiologist, I'm sort of semi-retired so I'm working sparingly now, intermittently, but I've been in the NHS since 1980 and a consultant since '93. In the last 20 years I've had experience in trying to innovate and my first job was in Whitehaven in Cumbria where we set up a new cardiac unit.

Nick Ferrari

Oh right? When was that sir? When would that have been?

Lance Forbat

Earlier in 95 to 2002 (NF "right OK") and then we did some innovative things with IT, transferred data across the Pennines with images, but *subsequent to* that I got interested in managing, *monitoring* people remotely having had some experience with what was then called the Docobo hub and I couldn't get interest in the Trust *subsequently* over the last two decades or the Cardiac Society in picking this up. Now some of it is because people wanted it evidence-based *no doubt*, but it's intuitively quite obvious if you're monitoring *someone* at home, which is now happening since COVID with the explosion of home *monitoring,* you can manage people and get them into hospital, delay admission, you can improve *their care before maybe* a procedure and you can get them out earlier or even prevent them going in. N*ow I,* the reason prompted this is an article on LinkedIn from Manchester where over 200 patients with cardiac conditions were monitored and it proved they improved care of them. And, of course, if you can get them out of hospital sooner or prevent them coming in that's one of the things that would affect the bed crisis. It's obviously not the whole story but I have examples of patients I've monitored: one lady who had multiple problems, not just heart problems but neurological problems *that I monitored her*e the six weeks in Australia through different climates, adjusting medication according to her blood pressure, ECG results and symptoms. And I've monitored and prevented patients from my home in Bristol, remotely for someone in Glasgow needing to go to hospital, prevention admissions and I've prevented delay of people coming out of hospital. I had you know only handfuls of tens of patients a go at a time, but these, these studies that have come out since have proved it. But trying to get someone interested, *unless you have got* a champion in the Trust and the funding there and even pilot studies that have been shown the benefit, say respiratory disease, *have gone for a period* and then the interest goes and the funds go and things stop and this has been...

<u>Nick Ferrari</u>
Why has it been so difficult to get someone to champion it do you imagine, Lance?

<u>Lance Forbat</u>
I think there's several things. People got to be on board with the concept, and a lot of people have their own little ideas and they're not willing to take advice from someone that is outside their little area or their specialty, or outside of their Trust. There may be some funding pressures obviously for the different things, but it's very difficult to introduce something as an individual. And unless you have a strong backing of your cohort of colleagues and even if you present something which is intuitively likely to make a difference *to the Cardiac Society or to someone,* or try your best, as an individual it's very difficult. And it's interesting how COVID has made it blossom because people were forced into having to follow the need. And I think the inertia, *you're tal*king about 20 years of potential inertia, and even if *we* said OK we haven't had *the full* evidence for last ten years, that's still a long lead time, time to get in innovation.

<u>Nick Ferrari</u>
It is. Lance, I must end it there because I had to get to the news headlines. Thank you for a. all your input and obviously from a professional perspective

and what you've achieved in the Trusts that you mentioned. Just before you go to the headlines, I'm going to leave you with some figures. …

Since Covid, that is in the last 2½ years, the NHS has had 16% lift in staff and 20 billion pounds more. Since Covid, let's just let that hang and go to news a minute late, 16% lift in staff and 20 billion pounds more, since Covid. So, it's not money, obviously. I don't even know if it's staff. Here's the last figure I will leave you with, the Health Think Tank, hugely respected, the Health Think Tank, the King's Fund. What do you suppose the cost to the NHS is each night caring for someone who could be discharged? 395 pounds. That is allowing for staff, costs, kit, doctors, rates, water, food, everything. That would almost certainly get you a night in a hotel such as the Ritz, the Dorchester or the Savoy. 395 quid what they don't have to spend because they can't get that person out. Isn't that the reality of what should be a true reform?"

Question Time in Bristol 12.02.26

I was in the audience for *Question Time*. On the panel were the Minister for Defence Readiness, Luke Pollard; the Conservative Shadow Science Minister, Ben Spencer; the Green MP, Ellie Chowns; and the Daily Mail columnist, Nadine Dorries. There were no questions on the NHS. I did, however, get an autograph from Fiona Bruce!

The first question was "Is Keir Starmer a lame duck?" I raised my hand, but neither my neighbour or I got a go. The second one was on colonisation of Britain and immigration and finally one on the increasing cost of housing in Bristol. They ran out of time for the fourth question, so we will never know. These were the questions I submitted:

1. How will the government ensure accountability of Trust managers who sack whistleblowers and change this toxic culture?
2. Will parliament give an amnesty to whistleblowers in the NHS with gagging clauses so truth outs and there is accountability for management who sacked them?
3. How can we trust the Freedom to Speak Up Guardian, when they are employed by the Trust and history tells us that whistleblowers are not protected?
4. Can money spent by Trusts making cases against whistleblowers, then sacking them, be recouped to compensate them for lost earnings?
5. Employment tribunals have no transcript of proceedings, ignore the destruction of evidence, and disadvantage whistleblowers. What can replace them that is fit for purpose?

Epilogue

There will no doubt be unanswered questions as to whom the author refers to in the parallel universe from his experience in the NHS. The readers can make their own judgement here and maybe can reflect on who they might be in their own experiences. The fate of the main characters will take many paths, but many are recently or currently employed in the highest positions within the NHS organisation and can easily be found.

Lessons learned from the actions of those in positions of power and the impact of the events in the parallel worlds they inhabit have yet to be fully realised. For those involved here, it would be disingenuous and quite wrong to react to my honest account by returning to the arguments of the organisations and individuals who were complicit in discrediting me in an attempt to protect their institution or their reputations as they did over 23 years ago, I believe with the clear intention to destroy my career (by rereferral to NCAA, GMC, wrongful sacking and a gagging clause). No doctor is faultless and learning from mistakes and having insight, knowing what is right and wrong makes a good doctor and it is proven civility saves lives.

Looking to the future I would hope those responsible for such misery and distress metered out to whistleblowers and their families like mine, will be brought to account. Should this not happen in the near future, then they must reflect on their consciences and live with the consequences that one day they most likely will be exposed publicly. Full compensation to those whose careers and lives were affected should be provided by the government, and I referred to this in my questions above. It may be a forlorn hope, but it should not replicate the delays and procrastination experienced by those who still suffer from Infected Blood or the Post Office scandals.

The culture within the NHS must change and good leaders who act with integrity and professionalism must be found who uphold the standards that we are as healthcare workers of all the professions involved are bound by Since 2014, the NHS has had to comply with a statutory duty of candour. It is essential the 'duty of candour' is protected, by providing robust support for those raising concerns, if the service is to be reformed for the benefit of patients and staff.

The transition from the situation I (for over a third of a century) and many have endured, to a better future, will require the political will for change, starting at the very top of government from the Prime Minister down and it should include the whole of the healthcare industry.

I hope readers will try to imagine themselves and their families in the situations I found myself, and try to 'walk in my shoes' to know how they would feel and react. What would you do?

Finally, I express my sincerest gratitude to my family and all those who supported me and I hope that all who read this book, whether whistleblowers, those afraid to speak up and all good people in positions of influence are encouraged to share their stories with their MP to make the changes needed.

Appendix

DOCTORS' EXPERIENCE: COMMON TACTICS USED BY EMPLOYERS
https://www.hcsa.com/media/399331/02-hcsa-speaking-up-on-safety-understanding-the-employers-playbook-electronic.pdf

HCSA has talked to doctors in this situation who found themselves put through an MHPS process. Their testimony exposed common symptoms and employer tactics used against those deemed a threat for speaking up.

EVIDENCE-GATHERING YOUR PRACTICE

You may be able to spot the signs that an evidence-gathering campaign is being run against you. This can include reviews of your electronic record notes and letters Crucial evidence may be altered and/or destroyed.

YOUR PRACTICE

You may find yourself under close observation or face interference with your treatment pathways

Colleagues may encourage other staff to make complaints about you, for example allegations of incompetence or outdated/inappropriate practice, over-investigation etc

You may face unnecessary referrals to Occupational Health/counselling with the suggestion that your judgement was flawed

You may be excluded and/or subjected to restrictions on your practice that you consider unreasonable and/or in breach of employer policy

There may be mismanagement of patients by others in order to "show you up" or trap you in some way.

YOUR COLLEAGUES

You may find yourself being watched by colleagues. This is particularly the case where there are potential conflicts of interest, either in direct relation to the safety issues you have raised or because of personal friendships with those connected to the issues

Staff that were supporting you may be threatened or punished

Those who are campaigning against you may try to exert influence with the medical director or their staff

You may encounter a lack of moral courage on the part of neutral colleagues who turn a blind eye, fail to offer support, or say they have no memory of incidents that they must have observed which would have assisted in your defence.

COMMON FLAWS IN THE MHPS PROCESS

ISSUES WITH ACCESS

HCSA and doctors who have been placed through MHPS have identified a number of common issues in employers' handling of the investigation process. If you are facing an MHPS investigation then it is important that you contact HCSA at the earliest opportunity. If you experience any of these issues then you should note them and inform the HCSA national officer who is assisting you. Just because there is a written MHPS policy, it doesn't mean your employer will follow it. Often this amounts to deliberate obstruction or abuse of the process.

ISSUES WITH FAIRNESS AND BIAS

Although in theory the MHPS process should be conducted fairly and involve neutral parties, unfortunately these checks and balances often do not exist in reality.

Doctors who have raised safety concerns and faced MHPS have reported issues including:

cont …

Failure of the medical director to apply rigorous impartial judgement

The designated board member being ineffective, disinterested or unresponsive

Unreasonable terms of reference

Issues which had previously been dealt with informally being resurrected and added to the terms of reference

Disproportionate treatment of you compared with fellow staff — for instance, minor technical breaches of policy being raised within the terms of reference when these are widely accepted when it comes to fellow colleagues

Malicious allegations made to the medical director included in the terms of reference

Unfair outcome letter following the investigation

Reliance on unfair reports written by an external expert

Failure to call an external expert as a witness, preventing the doctor from questioning them on their findings.

ISSUES WITH YOUR TREATMENT DURING AN INVESTIGATION

During an investigation it is common for an employer to take interim steps against a doctor. These may include being placed on restricted duties or being suspended from clinical practice. This creates another range of issues, such as:

A doctor being placed on restricted duties or being suspended without a satisfactory reason

Failure to review the restriction or suspension regularly

Failure to address requests from union or other representatives to lift restrictions or suspension.

Some of the issues commonly experienced include:

cont …

A meeting with the medical director is not held before the MHPS process is initiated

No letter is sent within seven days of meeting with the medical director

Terms of reference are changed or added to during the course of the investigation

Unreasonable delays or prolonging of your case

Inadequate time to prepare for your interview

Inadequate opportunity to present your case at interview, or not being listened to or treated neutrally

No opportunity to present further evidence following the investigation that would help to support your case

Being prevented from putting forward relevant witnesses

Failing to investigate a protected disclosure which was made during your interview

Misclassification of your case, for instance classifying it as conduct or SOSR (some other substantial reason) rather than capability

The case investigator failing to obtain all relevant evidence in terms of witnesses and documentation

Failure to clearly explain the allegations levelled at a doctor

Failure to examine disputed evidence prior to the hearing

Failure to provide notes of your interview to check before the investigation outcome letter is sent out.

THE DISCIPLINARY HEARING

What should happen. Should the case manager decide following investigation that an MHPS hearing should take place, there are a number of things which will happen next. If the process is being followed correctly by your employer, these should happen promptly within a set timeframe:

cont …

In general, the hearing should take place no more than 15 working days after the conclusion of the investigation

You should be informed at least five working days before the date of the hearing

All paperwork including your statement of case and any other evidence must be made available to all parties at least five working days before the date of the hearing. The same applies for the employer

All witnesses should be informed at least five working days before the hearing.

The panel will be made up of the hearing manager (senior clinician) and HR representation, as well as an expert in the clinical field, if required, who will advise but not take part in the decision-making process. You have the right to be accompanied by a trade union official or a workplace colleague.

HOW THE RULES ARE BENT AND WHAT TO QUERY

It's important to know what you might expect at a hearing in order to be able to prepare your-self. Here are a few of the things that doctors who have spoken up and subsequently faced at an MHPS hearing have reported:

What should and shouldn't happen during the disciplinary hearing process

ISSUES OF PROCESS

Failure to comply with the employer's hearing policy

Failure to address disputed evidence

Failure by the employer to call witnesses who made malicious allegations

Lack of opportunity to cross-examine the employer's witnesses

Inadequate time given to write your appeal

Failure to provide the details of an impartial person with no involvement in the original case to send the appeal to

Failure to forward the minutes or notes of the hearing in good time

Inaccurate minutes or notes. The employer may hire a barrister, while a doctor is supported by a trade union official or solicitor, or is representing themselves.

cont …

Biases among panel members or between the panel and witnesses which are not addressed. Your witnesses may be afraid to appear over potential reprisals by your employer. The employer's witnesses may lie openly under cross-examination, but the hearing manager states in their outcome letter that they "prefer" the evidence this witness has given an unfair outcome letter.

Records from my PalmV

'PIDA' flow sheet WHG

Text in black = neutral issues
Text in blue = bullying/harassment
C = complaint
Text in red = clinical governance/PIDA issues,
I = incident, Protected disclosure
My secretary away
My leave
Key events in Trust confidential summary of 10.10.02
Other confidential sources
NCAA process
Sent on leave by Trust
Wrongful dismissal

Date	Personal	My work issues	Trust response	Comments		
01.10.02		Met Trust & Avon HA.		Clinical governance Prelim' CHI		

Parliamentary and Health Service Report

Parliamentary and Health Service Ombudsman

Case reference: C-2002700
Complaint about: Ashford and St Peter's Hospitals NHS Foundation Trust (the Trust)
Complaint made by: Dr B and Dr E
Decision date: 5 September 2022

Our decision

1. We were sorry to hear Dr B and Dr E had concerns about the care their father received. We have identified some failings in the care the Trust provided during the first admission in 2018. This may have contributed to Mr N's need for a further hospital admission. It also caused Dr B and Dr E concern.

2. We have also identified a failing in the Trust's complaint handling. We understand the Trust has taken action to prevent some failings recurring. We are making recommendations as we consider there is more it should do to put things right.

3. We have not seen any failings in the care the Trust provided during Mr N's later admission. We are therefore partly upholding the complaint.

The complaint

4. Dr B and his sister, Dr E, complain about their father's admissions to the Trust from January to March 2018. During this time, they say the Trust did not: carry out medical and nursing assessments in a timely manner, follow management plans, carry out blood tests when requested, weigh their father, or maintain his dignity. They say there were repeated failures in care despite promises from staff and their concerns were ignored or dismissed.

5. Dr B and Dr E say the Trust denied there were failings in the care it provided. They feel it should have accepted checking their father's weight was vital to assess his fluid balance.

6. Dr B and Dr E are also concerned about the Trust's complaint handling. They say it took over a year to arrange an investigation and the consultant involved was not independent. They are unhappy the Trust did not ask for their input. They feel the investigation report failed to address their concerns objectively and included inaccuracies.

7. Dr B and Dr E believe their father's inpatient stay was prolonged to correct his condition and led to an accelerated deterioration in his general health. They believe this could have been prevented if the Trust had provided better care.

8. Dr B and Dr E were devastated by the events and say their family lost the opportunity to have quality time with Mr N. They have lost faith in the Trust and feel an urgent change in culture is needed. Dr B and Dr E would like the Trust to put service improvements in place.

Millbank Tower
Millbank
London SW1P 4QP

Enquiries: 0345 015 4033
Fax: 0300 061 4000
Email: phso.enquiries@ombudsman.org.uk
www.ombudsman.org.uk

Background
9. Mr N was 89 years old at the time of the events. He was taken to hospital by ambulance on 5 January 2018. During his admission, the Trust diagnosed him with acute kidney injury and sepsis.

10. Mr N had heart problems and had been taking diuretics (water tablets). The Trust stopped and restarted them during his admission. When it discharged Mr N on 18 January, it did not prescribe further diuretics.

11. Mr N returned to hospital on 15 February 2018 with chronic heart failure. The Trust discharged him on 8 March and he sadly died on 28 March. Dr B and Dr E complained to the Trust about the care it had provided. The Trust aimed to respond in May.

12. When Dr B contacted the Trust in June, it acknowledged there had been a delay in reviewing the complaint. In December 2018, the Trust concluded the reviewer it had appointed had not carried this out.

13. In March 2019, the Trust met with Dr B and appointed a clinician to carry out the independent review. It shared this with Dr B and Dr E in June 2019 and later met with them to discuss this.

14. The Trust acknowledged 'Mr N's admission on 15 February 2018 with acute exacerbation of chronic heart failure could have been potentially avoided at this stage. A combination of suboptimal discharge planning during admission in January 2018 and a lack of continuous community care led to a delayed start of oral diuretics at suboptimal dose.'

15. The Trust said there is no proven direct correlation between weight loss and fluid balance. Dr B and Dr E are healthcare professionals. They feel the Trust should have accepted checking their father's weight was vital to assess his fluid balance.

Evidence
16. In this investigation, we have considered the Trust's complaint file and clinical records from Mr N's admissions. We have also considered the information provided to us by Dr B and Dr E about the care their father received.

17. We also got advice from a consultant physician (our adviser) who has 15 years of experience. Our adviser is a geriatrician and suitably qualified to provide advice in this case.

18. We use relevant law, policy, guidance and standards to inform our thinking. This allows us to consider what should have happened. In this case we have referred to the following standards:

- Guidance from the General Medical Council (GMC) on Good Medical Practice, 2013. This sets out what it means to be a good doctor.
- National Institute for Health and Care Excellence (NICE) clinical guideline CG169, 'Acute kidney injury: prevention, detection and management', 2013.
- NICE guideline NG51, 'Sepsis: recognition, diagnosis and early management', 2016.
- NICE clinical guideline CG108, 'Chronic heart failure in adults: management', 2010.
- NICE clinical guideline CG187, 'Acute heart failure: diagnosis and management', 2014.
- Our Principles of Good Complaint Handling, 2009.

Findings

<u>Clinical care</u>

January admission

19. Dr B and Dr E are concerned about the Trust's assessment and management of their father. They feel there were failings in the care the Trust provided and say it only took action, like seeking input from cardiologists, when they raised concerns. They consider this was insufficient to prevent the deterioration in their father's health and his subsequent readmission.

20. National guidance from the GMC says doctors 'must adequately assess the patient's conditions, taking account of their history [...] and promptly provide or arrange suitable advice, investigations or treatment where necessary'. In line with this, the Trust should have assessed Mr N, put in place a management plan and arranged treatment.

21. When Mr N attended on 5 January, the Trust identified he had a urinary tract infection from his catheter, acute kidney injury and suspected sepsis. This was in addition to his heart problems and spinal stenosis.

22. Due to Mr N's clinical condition early in his admission, our adviser said the Trust would have been assessing him daily. This would have involved considering his fluid balance, his heart function, identifying oedema, and deciding on appropriate treatment. The Trust would be expected to document this and its findings clearly, in line with the GMC guidance.

23. The Trust should have identified and addressed the cause of Mr N's acute kidney injury, in line with the NICE guidance CG169. It should have treated the sepsis in line with the NICE guidance NG51. Based on the available information in Mr N's records, it appears this is what the Trust did.

24. The records also show the Trust arranged tests in line with the GMC guidance. Mr N's urea and creatinine levels decreased during his admission. This is evidence his renal (kidney)

function improved. His CRP levels, a marker of infection, decreased showing that the treatment for the infection was working.

25. Section 7.3 of the NICE guidance on chronic heart failure says 'all patients with chronic heart failure require monitoring. This monitoring should include:

- a clinical assessment of functional capacity, fluid status, cardiac rhythm (minimum of examining the pulse), cognitive status and nutritional status
- a review of medication, including need for changes and possible side effects
- serum urea, electrolytes, creatinine and eGFR

26. The guidance says more detailed monitoring will be required if the patient has significant comorbidity or if their condition has deteriorated since the previous review. The frequency of monitoring should depend on the clinical status and stability of the patient.

27. Before this admission, Mr N had been taking 80mg furosemide each morning and 40mg each afternoon. He was also taking spironolactone, another diuretic.

28. The Trust assessed Mr N's fluid balance and decided to stop diuretics temporarily after a consultant saw him on 6 January. They found he had an acute kidney injury so our adviser said this decision was in line with the GMC guidance, to address the cause of Mr N's problems.

29. The Trust appears to have assessed Mr N and the records noted he had:

- 6 January - no pedal oedema
- 7 January - swollen leg
- 8 January - leg oedema unchanged
- 10 January - no peripheral oedema
- 12 January - mild ankle oedema
- 13 January - mild ankle oedema on the right

30. After stopping the diuretics on 6 January, the Trust restarted Mr N on a smaller dose (40mg furosemide daily) on 14 January. Mr N received this dose until he was discharged on 18 January.

31. The Trust should have ensured Mr N was monitored in line with the NICE guidance to make sure the dose he was receiving was clinically effective. Based on the records and the clinical advice we received, there is no evidence this happened from 14 to 18 January. This was a failing.

32. There is no evidence the Trust planned to send Mr N home without diuretics so this should have been included on the discharge letter. This omission, without any evidence of clinical assessment or rationale for doing so, was a serious issue in this case. This is another failing.

33. Additionally, the Trust had already decided Mr N needed diuretics during the admission. Decision-making about this is not always straightforward, so it should not have been left to the GP. This too is a failing.

34. Our adviser explained the Trust should have established a dose of diuretic which was stable while Mr N was an inpatient. It should also have given instructions to the community team on how to supervise Mr N's ongoing management. Monitoring of weight is part of that.

35. It is difficult to know what the impact of the lack of monitoring was but the crisis which caused Mr N's February admission may have been avoided. We considered what the Trust has done to address this and whether it was in line with our Principles.

36. Our Principles say that public organisations should look for continuous improvement, and should use the lessons learnt from complaints to make sure they do not repeat maladministration or poor service.

37. The management and monitoring of diuretic therapy, correctly completing a discharge summary and proper handover to community teams on discharge are not things that should necessarily need a cardiologist to supervise directly. While we appreciate more intense cardiology input may have stopped these failings arising, we cannot say it was necessary.

38. The Trust has acknowledged Mr N's admission in February could have been potentially avoided if the discharge planning in January had been better. The Trust carried out an internal investigation into the lack of discharge medication (diuretics). This recommended discharge medication should be checked against the current drug chart.

39. In February 2019, the Trust published updated Discharge Guidance for patients with Heart Failure, with information about fluid intake, salt, weight, alcohol and symptoms. It includes information about local and national support groups and contact details for the Trust's Heart Failure Nurse.

40. The Trust appears to have broadly acted in line with our Principles. However, there is no indication it has identified the failing in monitoring Mr N when his diuretics were restarted. We are making recommendations to address this.

February admission

41. Dr B and Dr E are concerned the Trust does not accept it should have been checking their father's weight. Dr B says the Trust did not take careful steps to manage his father's fluid, he feels it just reacted to the input he provided.

Page 5 of 11

42. We considered section 1.3.5 of the NICE guidance on acute heart failure and sections 1.7.1 and 1.7.2 of its guidance on chronic heart failure. This reflects that diuretic therapy is used to treat patients with heart failure and weight should be closely monitored as part of this.

43. When Mr N returned in February, the Trust identified he was retaining fluid based on his clinical condition. His weight was around 15kg higher than it had been during his previous admission. Our adviser said the Trust should have assessed Mr N then prescribed diuretics. It did this and monitored him too. His weight dropped to around 70kg.

44. Our clinical adviser told us it is not unusual for the doses of diuretic therapy to need to be altered depending on how a patient responds to the treatment.

45. We have no way of determining now how those doses should have been altered, as this would depend on clinical assessment/examination as well as weight and blood results. Our adviser explained if a patient is losing weight too quickly, the Trust would be expected to consider prescribing extra fluids or reducing the dose of diuretic.

46. Patients or their families may have questions or concerns about the treatment. In these circumstances, the Trust should take their views into account. This is what the Trust did when Dr B expressed concerns that his father was dehydrated.

47. For comparison, Mr N weighed around 75kg when he attended in January. If a patient becomes too dry, their kidney function gets worse. Their diuretic medication can be changed accordingly.

48. Dr B and Dr E believe their father's health may not have deteriorated if the Trust had provided better care. Urea and creatinine levels are used for measuring kidney function. Mr N's urea levels should have been between 2.5 and 7.8 mmol/L. The normal range of creatinine is 64 to 104 µmol/L. His urea and creatinine levels on 24 February were 11.9 and 102 respectively.

49. Our adviser explained the management of a person with heart failure and fluid overload in hospital is dependent on repeated assessments. These include several factors (such as the weight, blood results, assessment of symptoms and clinical examination).

50. If the treatment is not working then the signs of fluid retention persist or worsen. If the diuretic is working too well then the person loses too much fluid and becomes dehydrated. This can cause its own symptoms and if severe can lead to stress on the kidneys and cause an acute kidney injury. Striking the balance between the two extremes is the aim.

51. Based on Mr N's clinical notes, when the Trust admitted him to hospital there were signs that he needed treatment with diuretics. Specifically, as well as his weight being higher that it had been previously there was a lot of oedema, crackles on the chest and a high JVP (which means the veins in the neck were fuller than they should be because of excess fluid).

52. Taking this into account, it was appropriate for the Trust to start diuretics. It gave Mr N 120mg of furosemide intravenously on 15 and 16 February. The clinical assessments on 17 February show the Trust had problems taking Mr N's daily weights as it needed a hoist to do them. When they were performed, the first weight on 17 February was 78.1kg.

53. Dr B told us his father's weight decreased by over 15kg from 16 to 19 February. We have not seen evidence of this in the Trust's records. The Trust reduced the dose of furosemide to 80mg given orally from 18 to 23 February, inclusive. Our adviser explained it is generally considered to be a bit less effective than if it is given intravenously.

54. The Trust then stopped furosemide between 23 and 26 February. It administered intravenous fluids on 23, 25 and 26 February. We understand Dr B's concern about whether the reduction in dose (and/or administration of intravenous fluids) should have been done earlier. This is difficult to answer, as we have no way of assessing Mr N in retrospect.

55. We can see Mr N's renal function (creatinine and urea) was improving throughout the admission, and his weight was relatively stable between 19 and 24 February. The renal function suggests any dehydration from the diuretic use was not severe enough to cause renal dysfunction (as Mr N's renal function improved during the time he was taking them).

56. We understand Dr B and Dr E's perspective. Based on the available information, we have not identified any failings in the care the Trust provided to Mr N in February. This is because the Trust was monitoring Mr N and adjusting the dose of diuretics. This was in line with the relevant guidance.

57. The complainants have described having to prompt the medical team to act to assess and adjust the diuretic doses in response to Mr N's changing clinical picture. The medical notes do not give that impression, and it seems that there was a difference of opinion at times about the correct course of action.

58. There is evidence that there were many discussions between the medical staff and Mr N's family. The actions taken may have been a considered addition to the management plan in response to the family's concerns. Alternatively, the family may have been directing the management, and without their input the changes would not have happened. Unfortunately, we cannot tell which is the case.

59. Dr B gave us an account of his interaction with one of the Trust's doctors who told him she was 'not confident' in managing heart failure. The management of heart failure is a core skill of a physician and geriatrician so we understand why he is concerned about that conversation. We recognise it is likely to have undermined his confidence in the medical team's management of the situation.

60. The entry from 23 February which outlines a plan of action to give extra fluids and hold the diuretics suggests that there was a plan to address Mr N's dehydration over the weekend of 24 and 25 February. We appreciate that the cardiology review which prompted that was requested by Dr B.

61. Unfortunately, the evidence we have does not enable us to know whether decisions on a particular day were appropriate or not. Our adviser said there are times when there is more than one reasonable course of action. For example, when deciding on whether to give intravenous fluids or just to encourage oral intake.

Complaint handling

62. Dr B and Dr E say the Trust took over a year to arrange an investigation and the consultant involved was not independent. They are unhappy the Trust did not ask for their input and feel the investigation report failed to address their concerns objectively or accurately.

63. Our Principles of Good Complaint Handling say organisations should deal with complaints promptly, avoiding unnecessary delay, and in line with published service standards where appropriate. We expect organisations to acknowledge the complaint, be clear about its timescales for responding, and keep the complainant regularly informed about progress.

64. The complaints correspondence shows Dr B complained in March 2018 and the Trust aimed to respond in May. When he chased this in June, the Trust acknowledged there had been a delay in reviewing the complaint. The Trust said this was due to human error. This delay is a failing.

65. It was only in December 2018 that the Trust concluded the reviewer it had appointed had not carried this out. The Trust appears to refer to this as an unavoidable delay but there does not appear to have been any correspondence with Dr B between June 2018 and January 2019. This was not in line with our Principles and is a failing.

66. The Trust has acknowledged the cardiologist who eventually reviewed Mr N's care provided sessional cardiology care to patients at the Trust. This clinician had not been involved in Mr N's care. The Trust said the two clinicians it had previously contacted to carry out the review were entirely independent of the Trust but neither could commit to completing this.

67. Our Principles say organisation should ask a member of staff who was not involved in the events leading to the complaint to review the case. With this in mind, we have not identified a failing in the decision to appoint a clinician who was not completely independent of the Trust.

68. Our Principles say organisations should consider the complainant's views to make sure they understand what the complaint is about. There was further correspondence between Dr B and the Trust following the report. He expressed that he had not been contacted during the review, his concerns were not fully addressed, and the report was not accurate.

69. It seems the Trust may have been satisfied it had all the information it needed from Dr B. When he raised concerns about the report, he set out his concerns about the staff and the discharge summary in 14 points.

70. The report is not structured in the same way so some points are addressed more holistically than others. The Trust agreed the report 'was not as detailed as it could have been'. There is a failing in communication during the complaints process. We recognise this contributed to Dr B and Dr E losing faith in the Trust.

71. We can see the Trust's review did not identify all of the failings we have identified. This does not fall so short of what we would expect that we would consider it a failing. We appreciate this shortcoming may add to Dr B and Dr E's concerns. We have considered what the Trust did following the complaint and hope this will provide some reassurance to them.

72. The Trust said it would consider standardising and providing simple guidelines for staff to follow, such as the Heart Failure Protocol. It told us it has updated many of the Cardiology documents on its intranet which is the main resource for policies, documents, referral forms and contact details.

73. The report author suggested the Trust should identify two main wards as hubs for patients with acute heart failure and to appoint an acute heart failure nurse. The Trust had a chronic heart failure nurse already and the intention was that these nurses would work between the two hub wards.

74. The Trust told us it had asked the Cardiology Consultants to consider this recommendation of a heart failure specialty ward outside of the recognised acute unit. The Trust told us it also planned to carry out a heart failure and cardiac specialist nurse/practitioner resource review to identify any gaps in resource provision and/or education.

75. The actions planned by the Trust appear appropriate to address the issues it identified. We are making recommendations to address the additional failings we have identified.

Recommendations

76. In considering our recommendations, we have referred to our 'Principles for Remedy'. These state that where poor service or maladministration has led to injustice or hardship, the organisation responsible should take steps to put things right.

77. Our Principles say that public organisations should look for continuous improvement, and should use the lessons learnt from complaints to make sure they do not repeat maladministration or poor service. We considered the action the Trust took following this complaint.

78. As we have explained, the Trust has already taken appropriate action to address some of the failings we have identified. If it has not already completed these actions, it should do so.

79. In line with our Principles, we recommend the Trust writes to Dr B and Dr E within six weeks of the date of this report to confirm which actions it has completed. It should also explain what action it will take, or has taken, to address its failure to monitor Mr N at the end of the January admission.

Findings leading to recommendations

What we are asking the Trust to do for Dr B and Dr E, to improve its services, and to improve its complaint handling:

Complaint issue	**What we found**	**What the organisation should do**	**What we need to see and when**
Clinical care - January admission, diuretics	There is no evidence the Trust monitored Mr N from 14 to 18 January to make sure the dose was effective. There is no evidence the Trust planned to send Mr N home without diuretics so this should have been included on the discharge letter.	We recommend the Trust writes to Dr B and Dr E to confirm which actions it has completed. It should also explain what action it will take, or has taken, to address its failure to monitor Mr N at the end of the January admission.	A copy of the letter sent to Dr B and Dr E. By: 17 October 2022
Complaint handling	There does not appear to have been any correspondence with Dr B between June 2018 and January 2019. The Trust acknowledged its report was not as detailed as it could have been.	The Trust should explain what action it will take, or has taken, to address complaints in an appropriate level of detail. It should include this within in its letter to Dr B and Dr E.	

"Do not judge me by my successes, judge me how many times I fell down and got back up again"

NELSON MANDELA

https://www.britannica.com/list/nelson-mandela-quotes